Birgit Makoschey

Investigations on efficacy and practical use of viral cattle vaccines

AF063495

Birgit Makoschey

Investigations on efficacy and practical use of viral cattle vaccines

Efficacy testing and practical application of viral cattle vaccines [Wirksamkeitsprüfung und praktische Anwendung viraler Rinderimpfstoffe]

Südwestdeutscher Verlag für Hochschulschriften

Imprint

Any brand names and product names mentioned in this book are subject to trademark, brand or patent protection and are trademarks or registered trademarks of their respective holders. The use of brand names, product names, common names, trade names, product descriptions etc. even without a particular marking in this work is in no way to be construed to mean that such names may be regarded as unrestricted in respect of trademark and brand protection legislation and could thus be used by anyone.

Publisher:
Südwestdeutscher Verlag für Hochschulschriften
is a trademark of
Dodo Books Indian Ocean Ltd., member of the OmniScriptum S.R.L Publishing group
str. A.Russo 15, of. 61, Chisinau-2068, Republic of Moldova Europe
Printed at: see last page
ISBN: 978-3-8381-2092-8

Zugl. / Approved by: Hannover, Tierärztliche Hochschule, Habilitation, 2010

Copyright © Birgit Makoschey
Copyright © 2010 Dodo Books Indian Ocean Ltd., member of the OmniScriptum S.R.L Publishing group

Table of contents

Table of contents 1

Abbreviations 2

List of used publications 3

A. Introduction 5
   Vaccines in veterinary medicine 5
      Live attenuated vaccines 5
      Inactivated vaccines 6
      Alternative approaches to vaccine development 7
      Production of Vaccines 8
   Viruses used in the studies described 9
      Bovine viral diarrhoea virus 9
      Infectious bovine rhinotracheitis virus 13
      Bovine respiratory syncytial virus 17
   Use of vaccines in control programs for viral cattle diseases in Europe 20

B. Definition of the problem 23

C. Results 25
   Challenge models for the experimental evaluation of vaccine efficacy 25
   Combined application of a live infectious bovine rhinotracheitis vaccine with other cattle vaccines 29
   Marker aspect of inactivated BVD vaccine 31
   Risk assessment for unintended immunisation of cattle by use of vaccines 34

D. Discussion 37
   Critical factors in the development of animal models for the evaluation of vaccine efficacy 37
   Effect of a live infectious bovine rhinotracheitis marker vaccine on the immune response to other cattle vaccines applied at the same time 41
   Evaluation of the marker vaccine concept for an inactivated bovine viral diarrhoea virus vaccine 42
   Risk assessment for unintended immunisation of cattle by use of vaccines 44

E. Summary 47

F. Zusammenfassung 49

G. References 51

Anhang 79

Abbreviations

BDV	Border disease virus
BRSV	Bovine respiratory syncytial virus
BTV	Bluetongue virus
BVDV	Bovine viral diarrhoea
cp	Cytopathic
CSF	Classical swine fever virus
ELSIA	Enzyme linked immunosorbent assay
F	BRSV fusion protein
FCS	Fetal calf serum
FMD	Foot and mouth disease
g	BoHV-1 glycoprotein
G	BRSV glycoprotein
GMP	Good manufacturing practice
IPB	Infectious balanoposthitis
IBR	Infectious bovine rhinotracheitis
IPV	Infectious pustular vulvovaginitis
M	BRSV matrix protein
MD	Mucosal disease
Mh	*Mannheimia haemolytica*
L	BRSV polymerase
ncp	Non-cytopathic
N	BRSV nucleoprotein
NS	Non-structural
NTR	Non-translated regions
P	BRSV phosphoprotein
PI	Persistently infected
PI3	Bovine parainfluenza type 3 virus
Pm	*Pasteurella multocida*

List of used publications

Makoschey, B.; Janssen, M.G.J.; Vrijenhoek, M.P.; Korsten, J.H.M. and van der Marel, P. (2001) An inactivated bovine virus diarrhoea virus (BVDV) type 1 vaccine affords clinical protection against BVDV type 2. *Vaccine* 19, 3261-3268

Makoschey, B., van Gelder, P.T., Keijsers, V. and Goovaerts, D. (2003) Bovine viral diarrhoea virus antigen in foetal calf serum batches and consequences of such contamination for vaccine production, *Biologicals*, 31, 203-208.

Makoschey, B.; Becher, P.; Janssen, M.G.J.; Orlich, M.; Thiel; H.-J. and Lütticken, D. (2004) Bovine viral diarrhea virus with deletions in the 5'-nontranslated region: reduction of replication in calves and induction of protective immunity. *Vaccine* 22, 3285-3294

Makoschey, B. and Beer, M. (2004) Assessment of the risk of transmission of vaccine viruses by using insufficiently cleaned injection devices. *The Veterinary Record*, 155, 563-564

Makoschey, B.; Chanter, N. and Reddick, D.A. (2006) Comprehensive protection against all important primary pathogens within the bovine respiratory disease complex by combination of two vaccines; *Der praktische Tierarzt* 87, 819-826

Álvarez, M.; Muñoz Bielsa, J.; Santos, L. and Makoschey, B. (2007) Compatibility of a live Infectious Bovine Rhinotracheitis (IBR) marker vaccine and an inactivated Bovine Viral Diarrhoea Virus (BVDV) vaccine. *Vaccine* 25, 6613 - 6617

Makoschey, B. and Beer, M. (2007) A live bovine herpesvirus-1 marker vaccine is not shed after intramuscular vaccination. *Berliner und Münchner Tierärztliche Wochenschrift*, 120, 480-482

Makoschey, B.; Sonnemans, D.; Muñoz Bielsa, J.; Franken, P.; Mars, M.; Santos, L. and Álvarez, M. (2007) Evaluation of the induction of NS3 specific BVDV antibodies using a commercial inactivated BVDV vaccine in immunization and challenge trials. *Vaccine* 25, 6140 - 6145

Kuijk. H.; Franken, P.; Mars, M.; bij de Weg, W. and Makoschey, B. (2008) Monitoring of a BVDV infection in a vaccinated herd by testing of milk for antibodies against NS3. *The Veterinary Record* 163; 482 - 484

List of used publications

Álvarez, M.; Donate, J. and Makoschey, B. Development of antibodies against non-structural proteins of the bovine viral diarrhoea virus in serum and milk samples from vaccinated animals. *Submitted*

Makoschey, B. and Janssen, M.G.J. Investigations on fetal infection models with bovine viral diarrhoea virus (BVDV). *Submitted*

van der Sluijs, M.T.W.; Kuhn, E.M. and Makoschey, B. A single vaccination with an inactivated bovine respiratory syncytial virus vaccine primes the cellular immune response in calves with maternal antibodies. *BMC Veterinary Research Accepted*

A. Introduction

Vaccines in veterinary medicine

The first successful use of a vaccine was in 1796 by Edward Jenner, who inoculated an 8-year-old boy with cowpox which subsequently protected the boy against challenge with Smallpox. Since then, vaccines have been widely used to control viral infectious diseases of humans and animals. In the case of humans and companion animals, vaccinology primarily focuses on the individual, while concern for the health of the herd is the main reason for vaccination of lifestock.
The first vaccines for veterinary use were live attenuated and one of the most successfully applied attenuated vaccines was the Plowright vaccine against rinderpest (Plowright & Ferris 1962). This vaccine has been instrumental in the near eradication of rinderpest. Another important achievement in the field of vaccinology was the development of the vaccine against foot and mouth disease (FMD), the first inactivated vaccine produced at industrial scale (Waldmann et al. 1937). More recently, the first vaccines allowing differentiation between infected and vaccinated animals (DIVA) have been generated (Van Oirschot 1999). After use of these marker vaccines the virus free status can be more rapidly granted to countries which have suffered disease incursion.
Vaccines for animals, have to be licensed by the relevant authorities. For licensing in member states of the European Community, EU regulations (EudraLex 2009) apply, while licensing of veterinary products in the United States is regulated in the Title 9 of the Code of Federal Regulations (C.F.R. 2009).
The vaccine manufacturer has to provide data to ensure that the vaccine is of adequate quality and purity, that it is safe and that it induces protection in the target species as claimed for the indication for which it is intended.

Live attenuated vaccines

Live attenuated virus vaccines make use of viruses that have lost their virulence while maintaining their ability to induce protective immunity against the virulent virus. The vaccine virus strains can be derived either from a virus naturally occuring in another animal species like Jenner's cowpox vaccine or they are generated by artificial attenuation. Louis Pasteur created the first artifically attenuated vaccine in 1884 by passaging the rabies virus in rabbits. This technique is also referred to as "lapinization". Other viruse have been attenuated by blind serial passages in heterologous tissues in cell culture or eggs. A different approach to attenuation of viruses is the generation of mutants either by chemical treatment, heating or spontaneous mutagenesis, which is an uncontrollable and random process. Therefore, these techniques seldomly lead to mutants which are sufficiently attenuated, while strongly immunogenic.
Advances in molecular biology, cell biology and immunology, especially the use of reverse genetics and recombination technology have allowed the rational design of vaccines. Genes coding for proteins involved in pathogenesis or immunomodulatory genes can be deleted, while protective antigens are retained in the genome, or even additional antigens are inserted.

Live attenuated vaccines can be administrated parenterally or through the natural route of infection, such as via nasal mucosa and mimic the infection at a local site. As the vaccine virus replicates in the vaccinated animal, virus proteins are expressed inside the cell. Thus they are presented in association with MHC Class I molecules which stimulate a cytotoxic T cell response. In general, live attenuated vaccines are able to induce an appropriate humoral and cell-mediated immune response shortly after vaccination with a long duration. After mucosal administration of the vaccine, a local immunity is developed in addition to the systemic immune response.

As production of live attenuated vaccines requires only minimal downstream processing and does not require adjuvants in the formulation, manufacturing costs are generally lower than for inactivated vaccines.

However, a general concern in the use of live attenuated vaccines may be the safety profile. The vaccine virus might potentially be genetically unstable or may cause problems due to residual virulence in immunocompromised hosts or during pregnancy. A recent example was the use of monovalent bluetongue virus (BTV) serotype 16 vaccine in Italy, in 2004, which caused undesirable effects, attributed to inadequate attenuation to European sheep (Monaco et al. 2006).

Inactivated vaccines

Inactivated vaccines typically contain a virulent field virus that has been subject to an inactivation treatment and an adjuvant to enhance the immunogenicity. The possibility to use field virus is particularly interesting in the case of those viruses, for which attempts to generate attenuated live vaccine viruses have failed or in situations where the generation of attenuated live vaccines is unfeasible due to time constraints. The new variants of influenza viruses or the outbreak of BTV serotype 8 in Europe in 2006 (Dercksen et al. 2007) are examples for such situations.

The use of virulent viruses for large scale vaccine production poses a certain risk for the environment as testified by the outbreak of FMD site in the UK in 2007 (Raleigh 2007) after the escape of the virus from a vaccine production site.

The efficacy of inactivated vaccines depends on a number of factors: i) the immunogenicity of the vaccine virus, ii) the amount of vaccine virus included in a vaccine dose and iii) the adjuvant.

Virus strains can vary with regards to their immunogenicity, especially in terms of the induction of a heterologous immune response (Hamers et al. 2001; Patel et al. 2005). Some agents used to inactivate the vaccine virus can destroy epitopes, which can negatively affect the immunogenicity of the virus.

The efficacy of the vaccine is a major consideration in the determination of the optimal amount of vaccine virus. Other factors are the induction of local or systemic adverse reactions, if these are dose dependant, and economical aspects.

Since the adjuvant effect of aluminium compounds was first described in 1926 (Glenny et al. 1926), they are the most widely used adjuvants, in both human and veterinary vaccines. It is generally accepted that alumium adjuvants are Th2 stimulators (Brewer et al. 1999), yet, the mechanisms that lead to the immunostimulating effect of aluminium compounds are still not fully understood. Initially it was proposed that the adsorption of the antigens to aluminium will delay their clearance from the injection site (Glenny et al. 1931), another possible mechanism is that adsorbed antigens may be presented to the immune system as

particles, which would favour their uptake by antigen presenting cells (Mannhalter et al. 1985).
Saponins are amphipathic glycosides extracted from the bark of *Quillaria saponaria*. They have been shown to stimulate a strong Th1 and Th2 response as well as cytotoxic T-lymphocyte (CTL) activity (Marciani 2003) and therefore were combined with aluminium in commercial cattle vaccines against BTV, FMD and the bovine respiratory syncytial virus (BRSV).
Apart from aluminium compounds, oil adjuvants, mainly water in oil formulations, wich induce a strong and long-term immunity, are the most commonly used adjuvants in veterinary vaccines (Herbert W.J. 1968). Multiphasic emulsions have also proved their efficacy as adjuvant as they can induce short- and long-term immune response with various antigens, with limited local reactions (Patil et al. 2002). However, the major disadvantage of multiphasic emulsions is their instability. Therefore, they are not widely used in commercial vaccines.
The application of most inactivated vaccines causes some local reactions at the injection site. The extent of these tissue reactions varies between adjuvants. Often, the severity of local reactions is correlated with the immunogenicity of the vaccine (Dupuis et al. 2009). A temporary increase in body temperature is the most commonly observed systemic adverse reaction to inactivated vaccines.
A new concept of marker vaccines has been applied in the modern generations of FMD vaccines, which contain purified vaccine viruses. Non-structural proteins (NS) are removed during the purification procedure. Therefore, vaccinated animals do not develop antibodies against NS, while such antibodies can be detected in animals that have been infected with the virus (Bruderer et al. 2004). Antibody enzyme linked immuno sorbent assays (ELISA) specific for NS are commercially available. The same principle has also been described for BTV (Barros et al. 2009). Studies to evaluate the same concept for inactivated bovine viral diarrhoea virus (BVDV) vaccines are described here.

Alternative approaches to vaccine development

The overall majority of commercial cattle viral vaccines are conventional live attenuated or inactivated vaccines. Alternative approaches are mainly followed if the conventional approach was unsuccessful. Subunit vaccines contain only one or a few antigens. They can either be prepared by purification of the antigen(s) from the virus (Nicholson 2009) or produced in a heterologous expression system (Zhang et al. 2000; Rai & Padh 2001; Mahmoud 2007; Mett et al. 2008). The latter has two major advantages: i) the respective pathogenic virus does not need to be cultured, ii) production yields in expression systems are often higher than for the pathogenic virus, allowing higher antigen doses in the vaccine. By nature, subunit vaccines are very pure. This advantage is more relevant for bacterial than for viral vaccines.
Vector vaccines combine some of the advantages of subunit vaccines with the advantages of live vaccines in terms of the presentation of the antigen to the immune system via the "natural" route (Brun et al. 2008). Recombinant pox viruses have been generated for vaccination against a number of different antigens (Plotkin et al. 1995).
Other vector systems have been based on a vaccine strain of a relevant virus in the target species in order to obtain a bi-valent or multivalent vaccine, like the bovine herpesvirus type 1 (BoHV-1) for cattle vaccines (Taylor et al. 1998) or the Newcastle virus for poultry vaccines (Veits et al. 2006).

Intradermal application of nucleic acids seemed a very effective way of presenting the antigens to the immune system (Van Drunen Littel-Van Den Hurk et al. 2001; Taylor et al. 2005). However, production of nucleic acids at industrial scale is not feasible until now and suitable intradermal injection devices for use in animals and particularly in life stock are not available.

Production of Vaccines

Industrial production of veterinary vaccines has evolved enormously since the times of the first FMD vaccines, when the vaccine virus was harvested from tongues of artificially infected cattle killed at the peak of clinical disease (Waldmann et al. 1937). Currently, production of veterinary vaccines must comply with the regulations of Good Manufacturing Practice (GMP) (CD 91/412/EEC 1991). All tests and processes as well as buildings and equipment must be validated and all steps of vaccine production have to be reported.

Vaccine production applies the seed-lot system according to which successive batches of a product are all derived from the same master seed lot.

Most if not all viral cattle vaccines are produced in cell culture either in roller bottles, or in so-called bioreactors (Gallegos et al. 1995; Moran 1999). The latter production system is preferred as it allows production of large batches with minimal handling. Both, adherent and suspension cell lines can be grown in the roller bottle system. By contrast, adherent cells have to grow on micro-carries to be cultured in bioreactors (Conceicao et al. 2007). Future developments will lead to the replacement of the traditional stainless stell bioreactors with single-use disposable formats.

Most virus production processes involve culture media that have to be supplemented with fetal calf serum (FCS). Due to the biology of the BVD virus and its high prevalence, FCS batches are often contaminated with BVDV. A protocol was developed to test FCS for contamination with BVDV (Makoschey et al. 2003). Using this test, most if not all commercial FCS batches are found to contain BVDV. According to European regulations, FCS has to be treated according to a validated method to inactivate potentially present BVDV (The European agency for the evaluation of medicinal products veterinary medicines and inspections 2002). The question, whether high levels of inactivated BVDV present in FCS used for vaccine production could cause a seroconversion in vaccinated animals was addressed (Makoschey et al. 2003) and the results are herein described.

Animal-component-free and chemically defined culture media for cells were developed to avoid any risk of contamination of vaccine batches with adventitious viruse originating from FCS (Makoschey et al. 2002b).

In case of non-cytopathic viruses, the cells are mechanically disrupted to release intracellular viruses. The vaccine virus is harvested by collecting the cell culture medium. Cell debris may be removed by centrifugation or filtration.

After harvest, live vaccines are mixed with stablizer. The resulting bulk vaccine might be stored frozen until filling into suitable vials and freeze-drying.

The virus inactivation is the most critical step in the production of inactivated vaccines. The first FMD vaccines were inactivated with formaldehyde (Waldmann et al. 1937). Formaldehyde cross-links chemical groups of the proteins in the outer virus membrane very efficiently, but the effect on the viral genome is les efficient, which may lead to residual infectivity in vaccine batches. Outbreaks of FMD in Europe in 1981 might have been caused by incompletely inactivated vaccines (Beck &

Strohmaier 1987). Arizidines like 2-bromoethylenamine hydrobromide (BEA) and its derivate binary ethylenimine (BEI) (Bahnemann 1990), as well as β-propiolactone have only minor effects on the protein, but interact directly with the nucleic acids (Blackburn & Besselaar 1991). The virucidal effect of ionizing irradiation is commonly applied to inactivate potential viral contaminations in FCS batches used for vaccine production, and has been used for the inactivation of experimental viral vaccines (Wiktor et al. 1972).

After the inactivation, down stream processing might be applied to purify the viral antigens.

The mixing of the antigen with the adjuvant is referred to as blending. In the case of aluminium adjuvants, the antigens are either precipitated by the aluminium or adsorbed onto pre-formed aluminium gels (Maschmann et al. 1931).

Oil adjuvants are prepared by mixing and stirring of the antigen, oil and a surfactant in order to obtain an emulsion (Jansen et al. 2006). The stability of the emulsion is critical for the stability of the vaccine.

Viruses used in the studies described

Bovine viral diarrhoea virus

The bovine viral diarrhoea virus has been isolated from cattle in all parts of the world. Some BVDV isolates are capable of infecting heterologous species (Liess & Moennig 1990; Paton 1995). In sheep, pulmonary lesions (Meehan et al. 1998) and in pigs leukopenia and thrombocytopenia have been described (Makoschey et al. 2002a). More recently, infection of white-tailed deer was reported (Passler et al. 2009). Two biotypes of the virus, cytopathic (cp) and non-cytopathic (ncp), are identifiable based on their lytic activity in *in vitro* cultures. Studies in cell culture suggest that the cytopathic effect may be the consequence of an activation of the intrinsic pathway of apoptosis (Grummer et al. 2002).

The genetic and antigenic differences between BVDV isolates (Hamers et al. 2001) lead to the recognition of two distinct BVDV species, BVDV-1 and BVDV-2 (Ridpath et al. 1994; Becher & Thiel 2002). BVDV-1 has been circulating in the cattle population around the world for several decades. By contrast, BVDV-2 was first recognized in North America and typing of BVDV isolates in samples submitted to the Oklahoma Animal Disease Diagnostic Laboratory revealed that 26% are BVDV-2 (Fulton et al. 2005b). In European countries, low prevalence of BVDV-2 are reported (Wolfmeyer et al. 1997; Letellier et al. 1999; Tajima et al. 2001; Hurtado et al. 2003). Some countries with high prevalence of BVDV-1 are even free of BVDV-2 (Stalder et al. 2005). Different subgenotypes of BVDV-1 and BVDV-2 predominate in different countries (Vilcek et al. 2005; Fulton et al. 2005b; Bachofen et al. 2008).

The seroprevalence in infected cattle herds can reach up to 100% and may vary between age groups within a herd (Mawhinney et al. 2007), with the highest prevalence in the multiparous cows (Luzzago et al. 1999).

The main route of BVDV transmission is via direct contact to a persistently infected (PI) animal (Ezanno et al. 2007). Virus spread from an acutely infected animal seems to be possible (Moen et al. 2005), probably even for a considerable duration (Collins et al. 2009), but by far less efficient than spread from a PI (Niskanen et al. 2000; Niskanen et al. 2002). Likewise, airborn transmission of BVDV has been

demonstrated under experimental conditions (Mars et al. 1999), but the epidemiological relevance is less important than the direct contact (Niskanen & Lindberg 2003).
The natural route of infection with BVDV is the oral or nasal route. Insemination with infected semen may also result in a systemic BVDV infection (Meyling & Jensen 1988; Rikula et al. 2008). After infection, the virus is spread via the blood and can be found in a wide range of host tissues, especially in case of virulent BVDV. As virus antigen is not generally associated with lesions in non-lymphoid tissues, tissue damage might not only be a function of viral replication but also be attributed to a reaction of the host (Tajima et al. 1999; Liebler-Tenorio et al. 2002).
BVDV strains differ in virulence (Ridpath et al. 2007) and post-natal infection with BVDV often passes unnoticed (Moerman et al. 1994). The degree of viremia during BVDV infection seems to be correlated with the severity of the disease (Walz et al. 2001).
Diarrhoea as clinical manifestation after infection with BVDV was first described by (Olafson et al. 1946) as a transmissible disease of cattle with a high morbidity and low mortality. This acute form of disease has also been reproduced by experimental infection of naïve cattle (Marshall et al. 1998; Odeon et al. 1999; Polak & Zmudzinski 2000; Ridpath et al. 2007).
A peracute form of BVDV infection was first described in the 1990s in Northern America and termed haemorrhagic syndrome referring to the clinical manifestation of massive bleeding (Rebhun et al. 1989; Corapi et al. 1990; Carman et al. 1998). (Ridpath et al. 1994). This disease has mainly been associated with BVDV-2 (Ridpath et al. 1994).
BVDV can infect white blood cells (Bruschke et al. 1998) and thus causes a depletion of B- and T-lymphocytes (Bolin et al. 1985). This may facilitate infections with secondary pathogens. BVDV might also play a role in the bovine respiratory disease complex (Thomas et al. 1977; Stott et al. 1980; Potgieter et al. 1985; Baule et al. 2001).
A distinct mechanism of acute BVDV pathogenesis is the negative effect on reproduction. Infection around the time of insemination might lead to lower conception rates (McGowan et al. 1993), probably caused by changes in estradiol and / or progesteron levels (Carlsson et al. 1989; Fray et al. 2000; McGowan et al. 2003).
If infection with BVDV occurs during pregnancy, the virus crosses the placenta and infects the fetus. Depending on the properties of the virus and more importantly the stage of gestation and the immunological competence of the fetus, this may lead to fetal death, malformation, persistent viremia of the calf, or the development of a BVDV specific immune response (Carlsson et al. 1989; Moennig & Liess 1995; Rüfenacht et al. 2001). Persistent infection has been described for ncp BVDV but there is no evidence that infection *in utero* with cytopathic virus results in a persisten viremia (Brownlie et al. 1989).
The PI calves are often born as clinically normal, but they may later in life succumb to mucosal disease (MD) (Malmquist 1968). MD had already been described in 1953 as a highly fatal disease of cattle with low morbidity characterized by extensive ulcerations on the mucosa of the gastrointestinal tract was described (Ramsey & Chivers 1953), but at that time the relation with BVDV was unknown. Further progress in the understanding of the pathogenesis of MD was made when Bronwlie and colleagues successfully reproduced MD by superinfection of persistently infected calves (Brownlie et al. 1984). Depending amongst others on the homology between the persistent and the superinfecting virus, animals will develop the early (in case of

high homology) or late onset form of MD (Fritzemeier et al. 1997; Loehr et al. 1998a; Loehr et al. 1998b). Under practical conditions, the latter might happen after vaccination of persistently infected calves with live BVDV vaccines containing a cp BVDV strain as the consequence of RNA recombination between the persisting and the vaccine virus strain (Becher et al. 2001). The antigenic diversity between the persistent virus and the superinfecting virus is not the only factor determining whether the animal develops early or late onset of MD. Comparative investigation of tissue alteration in cattle with early onset versus late onset of MD, revealed that macroscopic lesions were found in both forms of MD but cattle with the late onset form had milder lesions in the oral cavity while lesions in the intestinal tract were not only associated with the lymphatic tissue but frequently affected the mucosa outside. Moreover vascular lesions were observed in animals with late onset MD, but not with early onset (Liebler-Tenorio et al. 2000).

BVDV consists of 2 species, BVDV-1 and BVDV-2. Both are members of the genus *Pestivirus* within the family *Flaviviridae*. Closely related species within the genus *Pestivirus* are the classical swine fewer virus (CSFV) and the Border disease virus (BDV), and a tentative fifth species represented by a single strain isolated from a giraffe in Kenya more than 30 years ago (Becher et al. 1999). Within the species BVDV-1 and BVDV-2 different subgroups or subgenotypes are recognized.

Pestiviruses are enveloped single-stranded positive RNA viruses. The viral genome contains approximately 12.5 kb in one large open reading frame, flanked by 5' and 3' non-translated regions (NTR). The NTR of positive-strand RNA viruses are thought to contain important signals for translation, transcription, replication, and probably also packaging of viral genomes. Mutations in the NTR of BVDV and other positive-strand RNA viruses had lead to restricted growth *in vitro* and decreased virulence (Kuhn et al. 1992; Men et al. 1996; Topliff & Kelling 1998; Mandl et al. 1998; Becher et al. 2000).

The open reading frame is translated into a polyprotein of about 4000 amino acids. Co- and posttranslational processing of the polyprotein involve viral and cellular proteases and results in structural and non-structural proteins (Moennig & Plagemann 1992; Thiel 1996). Three viral glycoproteins (Erns, E1 and E2) are located in the viral envelope and the forth structural protein is the capsid protein (C). The Erns exhibits ribonuclease activity, which seems to be essential in the viral life cycle (Schneider et al. 1993). A second form of Erns is secreted into the environment of the infected cell and can be detected in the serum and plasma of infected animals (Kampa et al. 2007). E2 is the major target for BVDV neutralising antibodies (Donis et al. 1988) and probably involved in the initial binding of BVDV to the surface of permissive cells (Xue & Minocha 1993). Multiple attachment sites for BVD virus on bovine cells are proposed (Weiland et al. 1990; Schelp et al. 2000).

Investigations on the localization of BVDV proteins in infected cells revealed that the envelope glycoproteins Erns and E2 as well as the non-structural proteins NS2-3 and NS3 were closely associated with intracellular membranes, indicating that BVDV is released by budding into the cisternae of the endoplasmic reticulum (Grummer et al. 2001).

Among the non-structural proteins, the NS2-3 protein deserves special attention for two reasons: Firstly, because both the unprocessed NS2-3 and the NS3 protein are found in the cp biotype, while only NS2-3 can be detected after infection with ncp BVDV (Meyers & Thiel 1996). Analysis of cp/ncp virus pairs on the molecular level revealed that the respective cp strains arise by RNA recombination from ncp viruses (Tautz et al. 1998). The second particularity of NS2-3 is its high level of genetic

conservation. For this reason and because of its strong immunogenicity, most of the commercial BVDV antibody ELISA tests make use of the NS3 protein as a single protein or in combination with other viral proteins (Paton et al. 1991).
Transient infection with BVDV leads to a protective immunity. High serum levels of antibodies to BVDV can be detected from 14-28 days after infection onwards until up to three years after infection (Fredriksen et al. 1999). Colostral immunity is considered to protect at least partially against disease during the first months of live (Howard et al. 1989; Bolin & Ridpath 1995). Low titers can remain detectable until more than 6 months of live (Coria & McClurkin 1978; Bolin & Ridpath 1995).
There is evidence for the presence of BVDV specific CD4+ and CD8+ memory T-cells after acute infection (Glew & Howard 2001). However, CD4+ cells seem to be more important than CD8+ cells (Collen & Morrison 2000; Collen et al. 2002).
It is likely that an immune response is developed to most if not all structural and non-structural BVDV proteins. After natural infection, the E2 protein is the major target for neutralising antibodies (Potgieter 1995).
Infection studies of normal calves with homologous pairs of ncp and cp BVDV showed significant differences in both humoral and cell-mediated immune responses with higher neutralizing antibody titres being detected earlier with the ncp strain (Lambot et al. 1997).
On the other hand, acute infections with ncp BVDV result in immunosuppression. The mechanism behind this phenomenon has not been fully determined (Potgieter 1995; Brackenbury et al. 2003). Interestingly, ncp BVDV fails to induce interferon type I in cultured bovine macrophages whereas cytopathic biotypes readily trigger this response. Cells infected with ncp BVDV are also resistant to induction of interferon by double stranded RNA. It was proposed that this mechanism of suppressing a key element of the antiviral defence of the innate immune system may be essential for the establishment of persistent infection and immunotolerance (Peterhans et al. 2003). However, other studies confirmed that infection with ncp BVDV is associated with failure to induce type 1 interferon *in vitro* (Charleston et al. 2001) but also showed that alpha/beta and gamma interferons are induced by infection with ncp BVDV *in vivo* (Charleston et al. 2001; Charleston et al. 2002).
Different live and inactivated BVDV vaccines are currently applied and may be combined in a two step vaccination program (Moennig et al. 2005a). Both types of vaccines have been shown to elicit broad cross-reacting antibodies (Hamers et al. 2000; Patel et al. 2005) which are directed to numerous viral proteins. Several studies point to a correlation between the level of neutralising antibodies and protection (Howard et al. 1989; Bolin & Ridpath 1995; Beer et al. 2000). Moreover, a T-cell response is detected after vaccination with live vaccines and also some inactivated vaccines, depending on the adjuvant (Platt et al. 2006; Reber et al. 2006; Platt et al. 2008). Maternal antibody may block the humoral but not T-cell responses to BVDV vaccines (Ridpath et al. 2003; Endsley et al. 2003; Platt et al. 2009).
The primary aim of vaccination against BVDV is to prevent the congenital infection (Moennig et al. 2005b). General requirements for studies to demonstrate protection against transplacental infection are described in the relevant regulations for the EU (The European Directorate for the Quality of Medicines & Health Care 2009) and USA (United States Department of Agriculture 2002), however, standardized protocols are not available. Herein, studies are described to develop models for the testing of fetal protection.
Numerous alternative approaches BVDV vaccines have been followed in the past years:

Infection of mice with recombinant adenovirus expressing the E2 or the C protein of BVDV stimulated specific cellular and humoral immune responses (Elahi et al. 1999a; Elahi et al. 1999b). Similar results were obtained with recombinant vaccinia virus expressing E2 (Toth et al. 1999). Immunization with a recombinant equine herpesvirus type 1 expressing all four BVDV structural proteins protected calves against BVDV infection as judged by reduced viremia levels, decreased nasal shedding and maintenance of higher leukocyte counts (Rosas et al. 2007).
An E2 subunit vaccine produced in the baculovirus expression system induced seroconversion in mice (Ferrer et al. 2007) and protected sheep against fetal infection (Bruschke et al. 1997). More recently, E2 antigen expressed either in the baculovirus expression system or a mammalian cell expression system were compared for efficacy in terms of protection from viral challenge in cattle (Thomas et al. 2009). At a high dose, both preparation afforded a comparable level of protection, however, the efficacy of the baculovirus expressed E2 was greatly diminished when a reduced dose was tested.
Calves vaccinated with DNA coding for E2 showed no or only limited protection against BVDV challenge infection (Harpin et al. 1999), while results with a DNA prime – protein boost strategy were more promising (Liang et al. 2008).
The availability of an infectious BVDV cDNA clone allowed the engineering of viruses with defined modifications. BVDV mutants with deletions in the 5'-nontranslated region of the virus were reduced in their replication in calves and induced protective immunity (Makoschey et al. 2004). Also packaged replicons with deletions within the C, encoding region were capable of inducing a protective immune response (Reimann et al. 2007).

Infectious bovine rhinotracheitis virus

Infectious bovine rhinotracheitis (IBR) is the respiratory form of clinical manifestation after infection with the bovine herpesvirus 1 (BoHV-1). Infection with BoHV-1 can also affect the reproductive organ system leading to a condition termed infectious pustular vulvovaginitis (IPV) or infectious balanoposthitis (IBP).
IBR was first reported from outbreaks among dairy cattle in North America in the 1950s as a disease characterized by sudden onset, pyrexia, abrupt cessation of milk flow, salivation, dyspnoea, and severe inflammation of the upper respiratory tract including the trachea (Schroeder & Moys 1954). The IBR virus was isolated in 1956 (Madin 1956).
In Europe, the genital form of the disease was probably already observed in the 19th century and described as "coïtal vesicular exanthema" (Bläschenausschlag). The viral nature of the etiological agent was established in 1928 by Reisinger and Reimann (Reisinger & Reimann 1928). The respiratory form, IBR, only started to spread in Europe in the second half of the 20th century after importation of dairy cattle from North America.
Although IPV is usually not observed in respiratory outbreaks (and vice versa), occasionally the respiratory and the genital form occur simultaneously in herds (Kahrs & Smith 1965).
BoHV-1 is widely distributed among cattle in all continents and causes considerable economic damage not only due to disease but also due to trading restrictions. The virus can infect many wild life species as judged by the detection of BoHV-1 specific antibodies (Straub 1978).

After introduction of the virus in naïve herds the morbidity rate can reach 100% and depending on external factors mortality rates vary with maxima around 10% (Straub 1990).
The routes of BoHV-1 transmission within and between herds are different for the respiratory and the genital form of disease. Animals with IBR shed large amounts of virus with nasal and to a lesser extent occular discharge (van Engelenburg et al. 1995). The virus is mainly transmitted by inhalation of droplets containing infectious virus mainly through contact with an infected animal. Airborn transmission has been demonstrated under experimental conditions (Mars et al. 1999). Virus entry happens via the mucous membranes of the upper respiratory tract or the conjunctival epithelium. Infection via the mucous membranes of the genital tract takes place during mating and results in IPV/IBP.
After the primary infection, the virus spreads within the host via three different routes (Engels & Ackermann 1996): i) by cell-to-cell spread, ii) via the blood stream and iii) via the nervous system. It is via the latter route that the virus reaches the cells of the trigeminal ganglion (respiratory infection) or the sacral ganglion (genital infection), where it establishes a life-long latent infection (Pastoret et al. 1982). Latent carriers of the virus are clinically inapparent. Most of them are serologically positive for antibodies against BoHV-1, but there is evidence that some latent carriers can become seronegative (Hage et al. 1998). Moreover, administration of a live-attenuated vaccine in passively immunized calves resulted in BoHV-1 seronegative latent carriers (Lemaire et al. 2000a). Following immunosuppression caused by various factors including transport, calving and treatment with glucocorticoids, the latent virus can be reactivated. Reactivation generally passes clinically unnoticed but is associated with re-excretion of BoHV-1 and an anamnestic immune response.
The respiratory disease IBR is manifested by sudden onset of high fever, reduced appetite, increased respiration rate, and dyspnoea (Kahrs 2001). The animals have excess nasal and sometimes also occular discharge that is initially clear and later becomes mucopurulent. Hyperemia and reddening of the muzzle and nasal turbinates inspired the term "red nose disease". Necrotic lesions on the nasal mucosa are almost pathognomonic for IBR. Apart from the damage caused by the infection BoHV-1 or the host's immune reaction, BoHV-1 can play an important role in the respiratory disease complex, facilitating superinfections with other viruses or bacteria (Babiuk et al. 1988). The reduction in milk yield, that can be observed in the corse of an acute infection is probably related to the rise in temperature. When pregnant cattle are affected, abortions may occur between the 5th and 8th month of pregnancy up to 100 days after infection.
Cases of encephalitis with loos of coordination, hyperexcitation and depression have been reported in association with certain clinical forms of IBR, mainly in young calves. However, bovine encephalitis is more often caused by the closely related bovine herpesvirus 5 (BoHV-5) (Rissi et al. 2008).
Also the genital form of the disease starts with an increase in body temperature, but peak temperatures are usually lower than in IBR cases. Initially, small necrotic lesions become visible on the vulvar and vaginal mucosa. During the cause of the disease, the lesions enlarge and form plaques causing edema. Mucopurulent discharge is frequently observed. The clinical symptoms of IBP are similar to those described for IPV and limited to the preputial, penile and sometimes the distal portion of the urethral mucosa.
BoHV-1 is a member of the subfamily *Alphaherpesvirinae* within the family of *Herpesviridae*. According to antigenic and genomic characteristics, BoHV-1 is

subdivided into distinct but closely related subtypes, BoHV-1.1 and BoHV-1.2 (Metzler et al. 1986) and the latter further divided into 1.2a and 1.2b. Initially it was proposed that the two subtypes 1.1 and 1.2 may be cause distinct manifestations of disease, with BoHV-1.1 causing IBR and BoHV-1.2 being related to the genital form (Engels et al. 1992). The current understanding is that both subtypes are able to infect the respiratory and genital tract of cattle, however, it has been suggested that BoHV-1.1 is better adapted to the respiratory tract and BoHV-1.2 to the genital tract (Rijsewijk et al. 1999).

BoHV-1 is closely related to a number of other ruminant alphaherpesviruses: namely bovine herpesvirus 5, bubaline herpesvirus 1, caprine herpesvirus 1, cervid herpesviruses 1 and 2 and elk herpesvirus 1. These viruses share common antigenic properties (Thiry et al. 2006b) to the extend that BoHV-1 vaccines confer at least partial protection against BoHV-5 (Del Medico Zajac et al. 2006) and the caprine herpesvirus 1 (Thiry et al. 2007).

The cell-derived virus envelope contains virally encoded membrane proteins and a tegument protein. A capsid surrounds the genomic double stranded linear DNA consisting of approximately 135 kilo base pairs. The genome has the characteristics of a class D genome. It comprises two unique sequences, a unique long and a unique short sequence, of which the latter is flanked by inverted internal repeated and terminal repeated sequences. During DNA replication, both unique regions can flip-flop relative to the other unique region.

Ten BoHV-1 glycoproteins (g) have been characterized so far: gB, gC, gD, gE, gG, gI, gH, gK, gL, and gM (Robinson et al. 2008). The glycoproteins play an important role in the interaction with the virus host. Some glycoproteins like gC, gB and gD are indispensable for virus replication *in vitro*, they are referred to as essential. Others, the so called non-essential glycoproteins like gE can be deleted without abolishing the virus replication *in vitro*. The currently used IBR marker vaccines are based on gE deletion mutants of BoHV-1. Virus attachment to the cell surface is mediated by gB and/or gC (Li et al. 1995) that bind to cell surface structures like heparan sulphate. This low affinity binding is followed by stable binding of gD to specific cellular receptors (Campadelli-Fiume et al. 2000). The subsequent virus penetration occurs via fusion of the viral envelope with the cell membrane. At least four glycoproteins are involved in this process: gD (Liang et al. 1995), gB (Gerdts et al. 2000), as well as gH and gL that form a heterodimer. The capacity of BoHV-1 to spread directly from an infected to neighboring uninfected cells allows viral spread in the presence of neutralising antibodies. BoHV-1 glycoproteins gE and gG were shown to function independently from each other in cell-to-cell spread, because an additive effect on plaque formation was observed for a gE/gG double deletion mutant (Trapp et al. 2003). Recent studies suggest that gE is also required for anterograde transport of BoHV-1 from neuronal cell bodies in the trigeminal ganglion to their nerve processes (Brum et al. 2009).

After natural infection with BoHV-1, the first response of the immune system is the production of interferon alpha/beta. These cytokines can be detected within several hours after infection (Bielefeldt & Babiuk 1985). They might contribute to the early immunity after intranasal vaccination with a BoHV-1 live vaccines (Makoschey & Keil 2000b).

Only after a few days after infection the host develops a humoral and a cell mediated immune response (Engels & Ackermann 1996). Antibodies may either neutralize free virus or contribute to antibody-dependant cellular cytotoxicity (Tikoo et al. 1995). Antibodies directed against the glycoproteins involved in virus attachment or entry

(gB, gC, gD, gE) are critical in preventing infection (Babiuk et al. 1996). This defence mechanism has a major impact to control virus infectivity and spread after secondary infections or in case of reactivation. After natural infection, antibody response against BoHV-1 is longlasting (Kaashoek et al. 1996).
Once the infection is established, antibodies are of limited value in preventing direct cell-to-cell spread. Cell mediated immunity is thought to be involved in recovery from infection (Babiuk et al. 1996). The cell-mediated immune response to BoHV-1 infection includes macrophages, natural killer cells, gC and gD specific CD4+ T cells, and stimulation of cytotoxic T-lymphocyte activity (Hutchings et al. 1990b).
Maternal antibodies protect the calves against the clinical disease, but they do not prevent infection or the establishment of latency (Lemaire et al. 2000b). Moreover passive antibodies have been shown to negatively affect efficacy of a live vaccine (Patel & Shilleto 2005).
Like other viruses, also BoHV-1 applies mechanisms to evade the immune system. As discussed above, the most efficient ones are the establishment of latency and the direct cell-to-cell spread. Another mechanism of immune evasion that has been demonstrated is the inhibition of the proliferative response of peripheral blood mononuclear leukocytes to antigen (Hutchings et al. 1990a).
BoHV-1 causes a general immunosuppression in infected cattle, which often leads to secondary viral and bacterial infections in the context of the bovine respiratory disease complex (Bielefeldt & Babiuk 1985). BoHV-1 has been shown to infect CD4(+) T cells in cattle, leading to apoptosis and suppression of cell-mediated immunity (Winkler et al. 1999).
The first commercial vaccine against IBR virus was developed shortly after IBR was recognized as a viral disease (Kendric et al. 1956) and both, live and inactivated vaccines have been widely used in Europe in the US to control the disease. However, due to the particularity of BoHV-1 to establish latency, the application of vaccines in eradication programs was only possible after the development of the so called IBR marker vaccines, which contain a gE deletion mutant as vaccine strain (Kaashoek et al. 1994). After comparison of different deletion mutants, the gE deletion mutans were selected due to their favorable properties (Kaashoek et al. 1998). Since then, these so-called IBR marker vaccines are widely used, especially in those European Countries that have based their BoHV-1 control programs on the testing for antibodies against gE to detect infected animals. The efficacy of life IBR marker vaccines has been confirmed under field conditions in different countries (Mars et al. 2001; Makoschey et al. 2007b). Different vaccination schedules combining life and inactivated IBR marker vaccines have been compared under experimental conditions with favorable results for an intranasal vaccination with a life vaccine followed by the subcutaneous application of an inactivated vaccine (Kerkhofs et al. 2003).
Under experimental conditions recombination between wild-type and gE- vaccine virus was shown to produce a gE defective virus keeping part of the virulence of the parental wild-type virus (Muylkens et al. 2006; Thiry et al. 2006a). Despite large scale use of gE- vaccine viruses in different European countries, there are only very few reports on the possible emergence of such gE- wild type viruses under field conditions (Mars et al. 2000c; Dispas et al. 2003).
Any future BoHV-1 vaccine introduced in the European markets would have to comply with the gE marker approach. A gD subunit vaccine was tested in a large field trial in the Netherlands (Bosch et al. 1998) more than ten years ago, but until now, it has not been marketed, though it would comply with the gE antibody test. Moreover,

experimental data after DNA immunization with gD have been reported (**Petrini et al.** ; **van Drunen et al. 1998**).
Being a herpesvirus that grows well *in vitro*, BoHV-1 is an interesting candidate as backbone for vector vaccines. Studies have been performed with a recombinant gE negative BoHV-1 virus expressing the attachment protein of BRSV (Taylor et al. 1998) gave promising results. Insertion of genes coding for bovine cytokines did not further improve the efficacy of the BoHV-1 vaccine (König et al. 2003).

Bovine respiratory syncytial virus

The bovine respiratory syncytial virus (BRSV) is a major pathogen within the bovine respiratory disease complex. Cattle populations around the world are infected. Based on the antigenic differences between BRSV strains at least four subgroups (A, B, AB and an intermediate group) are defined and sequences are clustered according to geographic origin. Moreover, a continuous evolution has been recognized in isolates from countries where vaccination was widely used (Valarcher et al. 2000). The seroprevalence in infected herds can reach up to 95% (Collins et al. 1988). The disease is mainly seen in calves at the age between 3 to 4 and 12 months, after the maternal immunity is gone. Severe forms of the disease have also been reported in adult animals after the first introduction of the virus into a herd (Elvander 1996; Ellis et al. 1996b).
The disease can be seen during the whole year, but the number of outbreaks peaks in autumn and winter (Van der Poel et al. 1993) as a sharp decrease in temperature seem to trigger an outbreak (Mahin & Shimi 1982). BRSV maintains itself in a herd by airborne transmission (Mars et al. 1999) and regular subclinical re-infections of animals (Hägglund et al. 2006). Persistence of BRSV in cattle has been suggested (Van der Poel et al. 1997; Valarcher et al. 2001), but was never fully proved.
Animals become infected via their nasal mucosa. Replication of BRSV is restricted to cells of the respiratory tract (Viuff et al. 1996), with respiratory ciliated epithelial cells replicating BRSV much more efficiently than alveolar macrophages (Viuff et al. 2002). The virus spreads locally either by fusion of infected with neighboring cells or extracellularly via the mucus (Viuff et al. 2002).
The pathogenesis of BRSV is not yet fully understood. As infection of respiratory epithelial cells *in vivo* passes without obvious cytopathology (Zhang et al. 2002), tissue damage seems to be caused by the host's response to virus infection. BRSV infection induces an array of pro-inflammatory chemokines and cytokines that recruit neutrophils, macrophages and lymphocytes to the respiratory tract resulting in respiratory disease (Valarcher & Taylor 2007).
The severity of the disease depends on several factors: First of all, BRSV strains vary in their virulence. The list of animal factors that affect the clinical presentation of the disease include the age, the general immune status and specific immunity against BRSV, and the physiology of the respiratory tract of certain breeds like the Belgian Blue cattle (Lekeux et al. 1994). Finally, the disease can be exacerbated by co-infection with other respiratory pathogens such as bovine parainfluenza type 3 (PI3) virus or the bacteria *Mannheimia haemolytica* (*Mh*) and *Pasteurella multocida* (*Pm*). Mixed infections are common under field conditions (Assie et al. 2009).
BRSV and the human RSV are members of the subfamily *Pneumovirinae* within the family of *Paramyxoviridae*.

The viral genome consists of a negative-sense, non-segmented single stranded RNA genome of approximately 15,100 nucleotides. Ten mRNAs are transcribed from the genome and they are translated into 11 viral proteins, with the M2 coding for proteins M2.1 and M2.2. The genomic RNA together with the nucleoprotein (N) and the phosphoprotein (P) and the viral RNA-dependant polymerase protein (L) form the helical nucleocapsid. The latter is covered by a lipid envelope consisting of the host plasma membrane and three viral transmembrane surface glycoproteins: the attachment glycoprotein (G), the fusion protein (F) and the small hydrophobic protein (SH) (Collins et al. 2001). It is proposed that the matrix (M) protein forms the inner layer of the envelope and acts as transcriptional anti-terminator factor M2.1. The genome also encodes two non-structural proteins (NS1 and NS2) (Pastey & Samal 1995).

The glycoprotein G is responsible for the attachment of the virus to the cell, though non-essential as BRSV G deletion mutants were fully competent for multicycle growth in cell culture (Karger et al. 2001). Moreover, calves inoculated intranasally with BRSV deletion mutants were protection against subsequent challenge with wild type virus, indicating that this glycoprotein is dispensable for protection (Schmidt et al. 2002). On the other hand, calves vaccinated with a recombinant BoHV-1 virus or recombinant vaccinia virus expressing the BRSV G protein were also protected against BRSV challenge (Taylor et al. 1997; Taylor et al. 1998). The majority of the glycoprotein G is anchored in the membrane, and a minor proportion is secreted into the environment. A role in the immunopathogenesis after BRSV infection has been proposed for this secreted form of the G protein (Johnson & Graham 1999).

The fusion protein is essential in cell culture (Karger et al. 2001) and involved in the entry of the virus into the cell by fusion with the plasma membrane (Pastey & Samal 1997). Moreover, BRSV F causes the formation of syncytia by fusion of the membranes between infected and neighbouring uninfected cells, probably in association with glycoprotein G and the SH protein (Kahn et al. 1999). It has been shown that the F protein can inhibit the mitogen-induced proliferation of T-cells (Schlender et al. 2002). Upon cleavage of the F protein into 2 sub-units a small peptide with tachykinine type activity is released (Zimmer et al. 2003). This protein called virokinine might be responsible for the bronchoconstriction often observed in BRSV cases (Valarcher et al. 2006). The F2 subunit of human RSV was shown to determine the host cell specificity (Schlender et al. 2003).

Neutralizing antibodies induced by a recombinant BRSV that carries only the F protein, but neither the attachment protein G nor the SH protein, neutralized wild-type virus *in vitro* (Karger et al. 2001). Furthermore, a DNA vaccine encoding the F gene or recombinant vaccinia virus expressing the F protein both induced significant protection against BRSV infection in young calves (Taylor et al. 1997; Taylor et al. 2005). The results of all three studies indicate that this protein induces a strong antiviral immune response.

The SH protein is non-essential in cell culture, but SH deletion mutants of human RSV are attenuated in mice and chimpanzees (Bukreyev et al. 1997; Whitehead et al. 1999), probably due to the fact that the SH protein plays a role in establishing pulmonary infection (Valarcher & Taylor 2007). The actual function of this protein is currently unknown. For BRSV, the NS1 and NS2 genes are non-essential, though growth of BRSV deletion mutants lacking NS1, NS2 or both proteins is reduced in cell culture (Schlender et al. 2000). It has been demonstrated that NS1 and NS2 co-operatively inhibit the induction and the antiviral effect of interferons α and β (Schlender et al. 2000).

The protective immune response involves both, humoral and cell mediated immunity. BRSV infections are often recurrent, suggesting that the duration of clinical immunity following natural infection and vaccination may be short (Hall et al. 1991; Van der Poel et al. 1993). The cell mediated immunity was found to be essential for virus clearance following acute infection with CD8+ cytotoxic T lymphocytes (CTL) playing a dominant role in the recovery of calves from BRSV infection (Taylor et al. 1995). Other studies have supported these findings but also shown that cytotoxic T-cells are also involved in immunopathology and resulting tissue damage and functional disorders (Cannon et al. 1988). A number of viral proteins have been identified as target of the class I restricted CTL response, of which the M2, F and N seem to be the most important (Cherrie et al. 1992). CD4+ T cell epitopes were mapped on the F and G proteins of BRSV using synthetic peptides and lymphocytes from vaccinated, naturally infected or experimentally infected calves, in proliferation assays (Fogg et al. 2001). The CD4+ cells express a number of cytokines that are required for the cell-mediated immune response including IL-2 and IFN-γ, but others are involved in disease pathogenesis. The balance between the different cytokines produced by CD4+ T cells affects the outcome of the infection, both in terms of the efficiency of virus clearance and disease pathogenesis.

While the cell-mediated immunity is essential for virus clearance following acute infection, the antibody response plays a major role in the protection against re-infection. Targets for neutralizing antibodies have been identified on the glycoproteins G and F (Stott et al. 1986; Olmsted et al. 1986). Maternal antibodies were shown to reduce the incidence and severity of disease (Kimman et al. 1988).

Live attenuated and inactivated BRSV vaccines for active immunization are currently used in cattle husbandry practice. By contrast, despite the importance of HRSV infection, there are currently no licensed vaccines for prevention of this disease in humans. The reason for this discrepancy goes back to the 1960s, when a formalin-inactivated RSV vaccine not only failed to protect the children, but even exacerbated the disease upon subsequent infection (Kapikian et al. 1969; Kim et al. 1969). There are some reports on the reproduction of respiratory disease enhancement after experimental infection of cattle previously vaccinated with inactivated whole virus vaccines (Gershwin et al. 1998; Antonis et al. 2003). While millions of doses of such vaccines have been used in the field in the past 2 decades there are only very few reports on immunomediated enhancement of disease under field conditions (Schreiber et al. 2000; Larsen et al. 2001) and interestingly, the first documented case of apparent BRSV disease enhancement in cattle was following the use of a modified-live vaccine (Kimman et al. 1989). The mechanisms behind vaccine induced protection and immune-mediated enhancement are still not fully understood (Durbin & Durbin 2004; Openshaw & Tregoning 2005). It has been proposed that high levels of non-neutralising antibodies as opposed to relatively low levels of neutralising antibodies might enhance the disease, while cell-mediated immune mechanisms, including CD8+ cytolytic T lymphocytes, interferon-γ activity, or both, seem to be correlates of protective immunity (West et al. 1999a; West et al. 1999b). Comparing the experiences with different inactivated vaccines, it is difficult to draw general conclusions about the protective or disease-enhancing effect of an inactivated BRSV vaccine. Differences in adjuvant composition, or other differences in formulation, such as antigenic mass, the inactivation process, may be responsible for induction of disparate immune responses by 2 apparently similarly adjuvanted vaccines (Ellis et al. 2005). Thorough testing of vaccine candidates under controlled conditions is required prior to large scale use in the field.

As BRSV affects young calves after decline of the maternal antibodies, vaccination against BRSV should target calves in the first weeks of life, when maternal antibody levels are still reasonably high. It has been described, that passive immunity might interfere with the induction of an active immune response after vaccination (Kimman et al. 1987). Some vaccines are effective in very young calves, even in the presence of maternal antibodies (Mawhinney & Burrows 2005). Conceptionally, mucosal application of live attenuated vaccines should overcome the maternal immunity (Vangeel et al. 2005). Maternal immunization has been investigated as an alternate strategy to protect newborn caves from infection (Ellis et al. 1996a).

Commercially available BRSV vaccines are traditional live attenuated or full virus inactivated vaccines. A number of different approaches have been evaluated under experimental conditions, including a DNA vaccine encoding the F gene (Taylor et al. 2005) and recombinant BoHV-1 or vaccinia virus expressing the BRSV proteins (Taylor et al. 1997; Taylor et al. 1998; Antonis et al. 2007). The availability of cDNA clone for BRSV (Buchholz et al. 1999) allowed the generation of viruses with defined mutations. Viruses with deletions of single of multiple proteins have been generated (Schlender et al. 2000; Karger et al. 2001) and some of them have also been tested in calves (Schmidt et al. 2002). The use of expression products or deletion mutants as vaccines might have the potential for a marker vaccine.

Human RSV mutants with the G and F genes shifted to the promoter-proximal positions (G1F2) were shown to have increased virus replication *in vitro* without obvious effects on replication in the mouse, but with increased the antigen-specific immunogenicity of the virus as compared to parental RSV (Krempl et al. 2002). For BRSV G1F2 and G3F4 mutants have also been generated and tested in calves (U. Schmidt unpublished data).

The current knowledge on the evolution of BRSV strains should be taken into consideration in any new BRSV vaccine development (Valarcher et al. 2000).

Use of vaccines in control programs for viral cattle diseases in Europe

Control of infectious diseases is directed towards easing the impact of disease, with elimination of the agent, also referred to as eradication, as ultimate target.

Systemic vaccination has been applied to control the highly infectious viruses of rinderpest and FMD. In Germany rinderpest was eradicated in 1874 (Spinage 2004) and other European countries followed in the first half of the 20th Century. Also outside Europe, most countries are officially free of rinderpest and world wide eradication is expected to be completed within the coming years.

Germany achieved the status free of FMD in 1988 (World Organization for Animal Health 2009) and a non-vaccination policy was implemented in the EU in 1992 because of the estimated economic benefit of the respective sanitary status. Since then a number of outbreaks have been reported and stamping out was applied with the exception of the outbreak in The Netherlands in 2001, where ring-vaccination was performed, after adoption of the respective EU regulations. Vaccinated animals were slaughtered to re-gain the FMD-free status in due time (Bouma et al. 2003).

It is noteworthy, that both vaccines, the live attenuated vaccine against rinderpest as well as the vaccine against FMD were primarily developed to prevent disease upon infection with field virus, not to control the virus spread in a herd. By contrast, the aspect of controlling virus spread is a main quality criterium for current vaccines against IBR, BVD and more recently BTV.

Introduction

In a number of countries IBR and BVD have been successfully eradicated by strict sanitary measures without vaccination (van Oirschot 1999; Sandvik 2004; Ackermann & Engels 2006). Moreover, it has been reported that the prevalence of these viruses in individual herds may decrease due to a self-clearance process (Kampa et al. 2009). However, eradication without vaccination is only feasible and economically justified in countries with low cattle density and low prevalence.

Since 2004, voluntary BVDV control programs have been organized in nine states of the U.S. reflecting the recognition of BVD as an important and preventable problem (Van Campen 2009). The Commission of the European Union has funded a Thematic Network to control BVDV with the objective to provide advice on future management of the disease. The main conclusion of the network was that the technical tools and the knowledge needed for eradicating BVDV are at hand (European Thematic Network on Bovine Viral Diarrhoea Virus (BVDV) 2001). Three elements are common in large scale control schemes that EU Member States have already embarked on: biosecurity, elimination of PI animals and surveillance. The use of vaccines is considered an additional biosecurity measure advised in areas where the risk of introducing BVDV infection is high.

In Switzerland a BVD eradication program was initiated in 2009 (**Presi & Heim**). This program consists of testing the whole national cattle population for persistently infected animals in a short period. All PI animals will be slaughtered shortly after identification.

Voluntary certification programs for BVD control are ongoing in Brittany (France) (Joly et al. 2005), The Netherlands (Mars & Van Maanen 2005) and in preparation in Norfolk and Suffolk (UK) (Alston 2007). Although not prohibited, vaccination is not regulated within the Dutch or British certification programs. In Germany, a national BVDV regulation (Verordnung zum Schutz der Rinder vor einer Infektion mit dem Bovinen-Virusdiarrhoe-Virus (BVDV-Verordnung)) will come into effect in January 2011. According to this regulation, vaccination can be ordained or prohibited, depending on the epidemiological situation. Vaccination of female cattle has to be done according to the recommendations of the vaccine manufacturer in order to induce fetal protection (Bundesministerium für Ernährung 2008).

In the position paper of the EU netwerk for BVD control, the question is raised, whether vaccination interferes with the interpretation of serological test results. Herin, a number of studies are reported that adress different aspects of this question in relation to an inactivated commercial BVDV vaccine (**Makoschey et al. 2007a; Kuijk et al. 2008a; Álvarez et al. 2009**).

A related question is the one, whether high levels of inactivated BVDV present in FCS used for production of cattle vaccines could cause a seroconversion in vaccinated animals. This question was also addressed (Makoschey et al. 2003) and results are herein described.

Undoubtedly, IBR eradication has numerous benefits including an improved health status of the cattle herds and favorable trade conditions, however the costs e.g. for stamping out seemingly healthy virus carriers are also high (Ackermann & Engels 2006). The use of vaccines in systematic control programs for IBR was only possible after the introduction of the so-called IBR marker vaccines on the market in 1995 (Kaashoek et al. 1994). In the Netherlands, a national control program was initially started as obligatory program with half-yearly vaccination of cattle above 3 months of age. After an incident with BVDV contaminations in IBR marker vaccine batches (Falcone et al. 2000), the vaccination became voluntary. The seroprevalence for antibodies against glycoprotein E continues to decrease in The Netherlands.

In Germany, systematic control of IBR with use of the marker vaccine started in 1997. The progress differs considerably between Federal States. Some areas in Bavaria are officially recognized as free of BoHV-1 according to Art. 10 of the Council Directive 64/432/EEC (CD 64/432/EEC 1964), while almost half of the cattle population in other states is still BoHV-1 positive. Differing from The Netherlands, the target of the BoHV-1 eradication program in Germany is "seronegative for BoHV-1" including antibodies induced by vaccination. Under these circumstances, seroconversion of an animal after unintended exposure to vaccine virus has economical consequences for the farmer. Unintended exposure might occur after transmission of the vaccine virus to an unvaccinated in-contact animal. A study is described in which the question was investigated, whether live attenuated IBR marker vaccine virus is shed after intramuscular vaccination (Makoschey & Beer 2007). Another relevant situation might be the transmission of vaccine virus through unsufficiently cleaned injection devices. A risk analysis was performed (Makoschey & Beer 2004) and is described.

A third cattle virus that is currently subject to control programs in the EU is BTV. Mass vaccination campaigns against serotype 8 in 2008 with inactivated vaccines have considerably reduced the number of outbreaks as compared to 2007 (Kuijk et al. 2008b; Burgin et al. 2009; Conraths et al. 2009), with the exception of France, where the vaccination campaign was probably started too late in the areas with the most susceptible populations. Mandatory or voluntary vaccination campaigns against BTV 8 and other relevant serotypes were performed in 2009 in numerous countries in the EU.

In addition, vaccines against other economically important cattle viruses like the respiratory pathogens BRSV and PI3 as well as the parvo and corona viruses involved in neonatal diarrhoea are commonly applied. For all these viruses, vaccination is performed to prevent or reduce the clinical disease after infection with field virus. Reduction of virus spreading within or between herds is not a specific target of the vaccinations, but as the vaccines against these viruses reduce virus replication in the infected animal as well as virus excretion, they also reduce virus spreading.

B. Definition of the problem

The studies described herein are related to vaccines against three economically important cattle viruses, namely BVDV, BoHV-1 and BRSV. A proper evaluation of commercial vaccines is essential not only for licensing purposes, but also to advise the veterinarian on practical aspects for the use of these vaccines under field conditions.

Prior to licensing of a veterinary vaccine the safety and efficacy of a vaccine has to be established under controlled conditions. Prevention or reduction of clinical disease is an important criterium for vaccine efficacy. Any label claim with regards to protection against clinical disease has to be supported by study data, which requires suitable disease models. For this purpose, studies were performed with the three viruses to determine the virulence of potential challenge viruses, the challenge dose and procedure as well as the parameters that should be investigated in order to allow conclusions regarding protection.

A very practical question regarding the use of vaccines under field conditions is the possibility to combine vaccination protocols. This question is particularly relevant for IBR marker vaccines as programs to control BoHV-1 in a number of countries of the European Union apply voluntary or mandatory vaccination with IBR marker vaccines. Studies were performed to determine the immune response after combined application of a live IBR marker vaccine and an inactivated BVD vaccine or an inactivated combination vaccine against bovine respiratory disease.

Different possibilities for interference of vaccination with the interpretation of serological tests in BVDV and IBR disease control programs were investigated. A number of studies were performed to evaluate the question, whether an inactivated BVDV vaccine has properties of a marker vaccine when suitable tests are used for the detection of NS specific antibodies. In this context, both, serum and milk were evaluated as substrate.

As a distinct question, possible risks of the unintended immunisation by use of vaccines were studied. Some BoHV-1 and BVDV control programs apply monitoring of herds for antibodies to these viruses. Absence of these antibodies is required to achieve the status "free of BoHV-1" or "free of BVDV" respectively. Detection of such antibodies would lead to the loss of this high sanitary status and therefore has an important negative economical impact for the herd. Three different risk situations were investigated in this respect: i) induction of BVDV specific antibodies after immunization of cattle with a vaccine that contains non-infectious BVDV originating from the fetal calf serum used during vaccine production; ii) transmission of vaccine virus (e.g. the IBR marker vaccine virus) by use of insufficiently cleaned injection devices, and iii) shedding of IBR marker vaccine virus after intramuscular vaccination.

C. Results

Challenge models for the experimental evaluation of vaccine efficacy

Challenge models for BVDV, BoHV-1, and BRSV are presented. Most of the studies were actually performed to measure vaccine efficacy. These results are described as well, but the overall discussion will focus on the aspects related to the challenge models.

Makoschey, B.; Becher, P.; Janssen, M.G.J.; Orlich, M.; Thiel; H.-J., Lütticken, D. (2004) Bovine viral diarrhea virus with deletions in the 5'-nontranslated region: reduction of replication in calves and induction of protective immunity. *Vaccine* 22, 3285-3294

Two BVDV virus mutants (d2-31 and d5-57) with deletions in *cis* acting elements within the 5'-nontranslated region (NTR) were evaluated in calves to study their safety and their capacity to protect the animals against disease after infection with a heterologous BVDV-1 strain. The evaluation of a BVDV-1 wild type virus for it's suitability as challenge virus was a distinct objective in this study.

In order to study the safety of the mutants and their parent strain under "worst case" conditions, they were inoculated both intranasally and intramuscularly. While BVDV was re-isolated on two or more days from leukocytes of all calves infected with the parent strain, viremia was almost undetectable after infection with d5-57 and strongly reduced for mutant d2-31. The clinical presentation after infection with the parent was rather mild with some pyrexia and a slight drop in leukocyte counts. No clinical signs or decrease in leukocyte counts were observed after infection with either mutant.

Despite the differences in viremia, the course of neutralising antibodies induced by the mutants or their parent was very similar. BVDV neutralising antibodies were first detected one week after infection and titers continued to increase until the time of challenge infection with the heterologous BVDV-1 strain NY-1. After the challenge infection only a minor increase in antibody titers was determined.

After infection with the BVD-1 strain NY-1, BVDV was re-isolated on three or more days from leukocytes of all three calves that were naïve at the time of challenge. By contrast all samples taken from animals that had been previously infected with one of the mutants or their parent were tested negative for BVDV.

Taken the absence of viremia after challenge infection and the lack of a clear anamnestic response together they are indicative for a sterile immunity in the three groups that had been infected before with the mutants or their parent.

Unfortunately only one out of three animals that were naïve at the time of infection with strain NY-1 showed clear signs of respiratory disease including an elevated body temperature. Very mild respiratory signs were observed in the two other animals of this group. The only obvious effects of infection with NY-1 in naïve animals were the decrease in leukocyte counts and to a lesser extent also in lymphocyte counts. Both, the leukocyte counts and the lymphocyte counts remained within the physiological range in the animals that had been previously infected with one of the mutants or their parent. Due to the fact that parent virus was not pathogenic, no conclusions are possible with regards to the attenuation of the mutants. By contrast, it can be concluded that both mutants confer protection as judged by the serological, virological and haematological findings after challenge infection.

Makoschey, B.; Janssen, M.G.J.; Vrijenhoek, M.P.; Korsten, J.H.M.; van der Marel, P. (2001) **An inactivated bovine virus diarrhoea virus (BVDV) type 1 vaccine affords clinical protection against BVDV type 2.** *Vaccine* 19, 3261-3268

After the first reports on an apparently new clinical manifestation of BVDV infection, the so-called haemorrhagic syndrome, the question was raised whether signs of acute BVDV-2 infection including symptoms of haemorrhagic disease can be reproduced under experimental conditions in calves at 20 weeks of age. Moreover, it should be investigated whether an inactivated BVDV-1 vaccine protects against this disease. One group of calves was vaccinated twice with an inactivated BVDV-1 vaccine at the age of 12 and 16 weeks. Four weeks after the second vaccination they were infected intravenously and intranasally with a pair of ncp and cp virus of the BVDV-2 strain GiI that had been isolated originally from a calf with haemorrhagic symptoms. Five age matched unvaccinated calves were infected similarly at the same time.

The successful infection of the animals was confirmed by the re-isolation of BVDV from blood cells of all unvaccinated animals. BVDV was also re-isolated from blood cells of three vaccinated animals.

Four out of five unvaccinated animals developed diarrhoea after challenge infection, while only mild respiratory signs were recorded for the vaccinated calves and uninfected control animals. The unvaccinated animals developed a biphasic pyrexia with peak temperatures up to 41°C at two and seven days after infection. The temperature curves of the vaccinated animals followed a similar pattern but the average temperatures were lower than for the unvaccinated animals. Throughout the whole study, the temperatures of the unvaccinated animals remained within the physiological range.

The unvaccinated animals displayed a dramatic drop in leukocyte counts within the first week after infection. Normal values were only reached at more than two weeks after infection. The leukocyte counts of the vaccinated animals also decreased, though to a lesser extent than in the unvaccinated animals, and the animals recovered much quicker.

The thrombocyte counts were monitored as thrombocytopenia was reported from cases of haemorrhagic disease after infection with BVDV-2. Also in this study, unvaccinated animals experienced a dramatic drop in thrombocyte counts, followed by an increase beyond normal levels. Values within the normal reference range were only reached at three weeks after infection. By contrast, animals that were vaccinated prior to challenge infection showed only a slight decrease in thrombocyte counts and values had normalized within two weeks after infection.

The different levels of thrombocytopenia in the unvaccinated and vaccinated animals were reflected in the findings during autopsy. Clotting of the blood was impaired in two unvaccinated animals and megakaryocytosis was observed.

Being the predominant findings, erosions and petechial haemorrhages throughout the gastro-intestinal were less numerous and severe in the vaccinated animals. Crypt necrosis and formation of micro-abscesses were found upon histological examination of these lesions.

Severe lymphatic depletion in both, central in peripheral lymphatic tissues was seen in unvaccinated calves at 9 days after infection with BVDV-2 GiI, while the lymphatic organs of vaccinated animals were normal at the same time point.

Makoschey, B.; Janssen, M.G.J. Investigations on fetal infection models with bovine viral diarrhoea virus (BVDV). *Submitted*

In the case of BVDV, prevention of fetal infection is the primary goal for vaccination besides the protection against clinical disease. Studies were performed to develop models to test fetal protection. Firstly, the possibility of dual challenge with BVDV-1 and BVDV-2 was evaluated and in a separate approach the transmission of BVDV-2 from a persistently infected calf to in-contact animals was investigated.

Two studies were performed in pregnant heifers to determine whether concurrent inoculation of one BVDV-2 and one BVDV-2 strain, separately into either nostril results in fetal infection with both viruses.

Leukocytes were tested for infectious BVDV by co-culture with a suitable cell line. After infection, BVDV was re-isolated from leukocytes of all heifers on at least one day, with peak levels around seven or eight days after infection and a duration until two weeks after infection. One out of three samples on which specific PCR was performed was found positive for BVDV-1 and BVDV-2, while only BVDV-1 was detected in the two others.

All heifers developed mild to moderate signs of respiratory disease at varying degree after infection with the two BVDV strains. The numbers of circulating leukocytes decreased after the infection with BVDV and recovered only after more than two weeks post infection in the first study, while recovery occurred within less than two weeks in the second study.

The heifers experienced a drop in platelet counts starting four to five days after infection with BVDV. In the first study, the platelet counts remained at a low level for several days and normal values were only reached at three weeks after infection. In the second study, the recovery took place within a few days.

As studying fetal infection with BVDV was the main objective of the studies, the outcome of the pregnancy and the viremia in calves were of major interest: With the exception of one heifer in the first study that aborted six weeks after the infection with BVDV all pregnancies resulted in the birth of clinically normal calves. One cow in the second study gave birth to twins, all other pregnancies were single calves. BVDV could be re-isolated from pre-colostral blood samples with the exception of one calf, of which the sample was cytotoxic and therefore, not suitable for passaging in cell culture. BVDV could also be isolated from the organ samples of the aborted fetus. Dual infection with BVDV-1 and BVDV-2 was detected by specific PCR in the samples obtained from the aborted fetus. By contrast, only BVDV-2 was detected in all blood samples from the calves in the second study.

As dual fetal infection could not consistently be achieved after concurrent inoculation with BVDV-1 and BVDV-2 a separate study was performed to investigate the possibility of BVDV-2 challenge by contact with a persistently infected animal. Four susceptible heifers were housed as a group adjacent to a pen in which a calf persistently infected with BVDV-2 was placed. BVDV infection in the heifers was monitored by testing weekly blood samples for antibodies. Transmission of BVDV-2 from a PI animal was found to be fast and efficient as three out of four sentinels developed antibodies against BVDV already within three weeks and the fourth animal seroconverted during the following week. Thus the results demonstrate that BVDV-2 virus transmission is very efficient if the animals have direct contact, even if they are separated by a fence. None of the in-contact animals developed clinical disease after BVDV infection.

Makoschey, B.; Chanter, N.; Reddick, D.A. (2006) Comprehensive protection against all important primary pathogens within the bovine respiratory disease complex by combination of two vaccines; *Der praktische Tierarzt* **87, 819-826**

The efficacy after concurrent application of a live IBR marker vaccine and an inactivated combination vaccine against respiratory disease containing BRSV - bovine parainfluenza type 3 virus (PI3) and Mannheimia haemolytica (*Mh*) antigens should be demonstrated. Separate challenge studies were performed with the four pathogens. In the context of the development of challenge models, only the results of the infection study with BoHV-1 are summarized below. The studies with BRSV, PI3 and *Mh* challenge will be presented in the section addressing the combined application of vaccines.

The BoHV-1 challenge study was performed in calves at the age of about 2 weeks without maternal antibodies. Two groups each were vaccinated intranasally (IN) and intramuscularly (IM) with a live BoHV-1 marker vaccine. At the same time, one IN group and one IM group received one dose of the inactivated BRSV-PI3-*Mh* combination vaccine via the SC route in order to study possible effects of a combined application of the two vaccines. Antibodies against BoHV-1 were measured from two weeks after the single vaccination onwards in all four vaccinated groups with no differences between single and concurrent use of the vaccine.

Four weeks after the vaccination all animals were challenged IN with a virulent BoHV-1 field isolate.

BoHV-1 challenge virus was recovered at high titers from nasal discharge of unvaccinated animals. Both, average as well as maximum BoHV-1 titers were significantly lower after vaccination as compared to the unvaccinated group.

After challenge, clinical signs of respiratory disease like coughing, nasal discharge and erosions of the mucosa were observed in all unvaccinated animals. Moreover, the unvaccinated animals developed pyrexia. The clinical signs after challenge of vaccinated animals were clearly milder and the body temperatures remained within physiological limits.

van der Sluijs, M.T.W.; Kuhn, E.M.; Makoschey, B. A single vaccination with an inactivated bovine respiratory syncytial virus vaccine primes the cellular immune response in calves with maternal antibodies. *BMC Veterinary Research* *Accepted*

As clinical disease after infection with BRSV is typically observed in young calves, vaccination against this virus should start at an early age. Given the high prevalence of BRSV in Germany and most other cattle industries, most calves will have maternal antibodies. While these antibodies do not prevent disease, they might negatively interfere with the vaccination. Therefore, efficacy of BRSV vaccines has to be demonstrated in calves with maternal antibodies. Clinical signs after infection with BRSV under laboratory conditions arer often milder than under field conditions. The virulence of a BRSV field isolate was tested after challenge by aerosolization. Different parameters were studied to judge the virulence of the virus as well as the protection after single application of an inactivated BRSV - PI3 – *Mh* combination vaccine.

As expected the single vaccination, did not have an effect on the decline of the BRSV-specific maternal antibodies. However, results of lymphocyte activation assays

in which specific stimulation was detected by quantification of Interferon γ indicated that the cellular immune system was primed by the single dose of the vaccine.
After BRSV infection, there were only minor clinical signs observed and the body temperatures remained within the physiological limits. Likewise, no or only minor lesions were detected in the lungs of most calves in both groups. Only one unvaccinated animal had considerable lung pathology with 50 or 70% of the right apical lobe affected and the medial lobe consolidated. The lung of one vaccinated animal showed dark red consolidation of 10-25% of the medial and apical lung lobes. Syncytial cells, which are characteristic for BRSV infection were present in two vaccinated animals and suspected in one control animal.
BRSV could be re-isolated from nasal swab samples from three out of four unvaccinated animals during two or three days. The maximum titers and the number of days, when virus was excreted was significantly lower in the vaccinated group as compared to the unvaccinated group.
Infection with BRSV was confirmed in tissue samples taken from the respiratory tract of all animals except one vaccinated animal. However, the number of positive samples was higher in the unvaccinated group than in the vaccinates.
The lung wash fluid of two animals, one from the unvaccinated and one from the vaccinated group was found positive for BRSV, all other samples were negative.

Combined application of a live infectious bovine rhinotracheitis vaccine with other cattle vaccines

Álvarez, M.; Muñoz Bielsa, J.; Santos, L.; Makoschey, B. (2007) Compatibility of a Live Infectious Bovine Rhinotracheitis (IBR) Marker Vaccine and an Inactivated Bovine Viral Diarrhoea Virus (BVDV). *Vaccine* **25, 6613 - 6617**

Different combined vaccination schedules for a live IBR marker vaccine and an inactivated BVDV were compared with respect to the induction of BoHV-1 and BVDV neutralising antibodies. The study was performed in 6 to 8 months old heifers, all of them were seronegative for BoHV-1 and BVDV at the start of the study. The animals were vaccinated three times, with an interval of 4 weeks between the first and second vaccination and an interval of 6 months between the second and third vaccination.
For simultaneous application of the two vaccines, the inactivated BVD vaccine was used to reconstitute the freeze-dried live vaccine and administered as one injection. For concurrent application, the two vaccines were applied at the same time but as two injections at separate injection sites.
All animals that were only vaccinated with the BVDV vaccine remained seronegative for BoHV-1 neutralising antibodies throughout the study. Vaccination with the live IBR marker vaccine induced BoHV-1 neutralising antibodies in all animals. The antibody titres further increased in those animals that received a second dose. Simultaneous application of the BVDV vaccine together with the IBR marker vaccine resulted in significantly higher BoHV-1 neutralising antibodies than application of the IBR marker vaccine alone.
The animals that were only vaccinated with the live IBR marker vaccine remained seronegative for BVDV until the end of the study. After the first dose of the inactivated BVDV vaccine, neutralising antibodies were detected in some of the animals, while the remaining animals in the respective groups developed a good

antibody response after the second vaccination. BVDV antibody titres were not negatively affected when the IBR marker vaccine was applied simultaneously at the first or second dose of the BVD basic vaccination and / or at the re-vaccination. Yet, antibody titres were significantly lower when the IBR marker vaccine was given simultaneously for the first and second dose of the BVDV basic vaccination. Concurrent application of the two vaccines at the first, second and third vaccination induced similar antibody titres than the BVD vaccine alone.

Makoschey, B.; Chanter, N.; Reddick, D.A. (2006) Comprehensive protection against all important primary pathogens within the bovine respiratory disease complex by combination of two vaccines; *Der praktische Tierarzt* **87, 819-826**

Different challenge studies were performed to demonstrate the efficacy of the individual vaccines after concurrent application of a live IBR marker vaccine and an inactivated BRSV-PI3-*Mh* combination vaccine. The results of the BoHV-1 challenge study are addressed in the context of the development of challenge models (see above). Here, the studies with BRSV, PI3 and *Mh* challenge are presented.
Two studies were performed in colostrum deprived calves. Animals were challenged sequentially with the two viruses in the first study and protection against challenge infection with *Mh* was measured in the second study.
In the first study, one group of ten calves at the age of two weeks was vaccinated subcutaneously (SC) with the inactivated BRSV-PI3-*Mh* combination vaccine and at the same time with the live IBR marker vaccine, both IN and IM. A second group of nine calves was only vaccinated with the inactivated combination vaccine. Vaccination with the inactivated combination vaccine was repeated four weeks later. Both vaccinated groups together with an unvaccinated control group were first challenge infected with BRSV at 3 weeks after the second vaccination with the inactivated BRSV-PI3-*Mh* vaccine and five weeks later with PI3.
There were no differences in antibody response after vaccination and challenge between the two vaccinated groups.
As the unvaccinated control animals developed few if any clinical signs that could be directly attributed to the BRSV and PI3 challenges no conclusions regarding protection against clinical sings after infection with the two viruses were possible.
Concurrent application of the live IBR marker vaccine did not affect efficacy of the inactivated combination vaccine with regards to protection against shedding of BRSV and PI3 as demonstrated by the shorter duration, delayed onset, fewer numbers of animals shedding virus and lower virus titres being recovered.
For the *Mh* challenge study, three groups of were vaccinated with the inactivated combination vaccine at the age of 2 and 6 weeks. At the time of the first vaccination the live IBR marker vaccine was applied as well in two of the three groups, one group was vaccinated IM and the second IM. A fourth group was kept as unvaccinated controls. Two weeks after the second vaccination, all animals were challenged intratracheally with *Mh*.
There were no differences in *Mh* antibody response after vaccination between the three vaccinated groups. Due to the study design, no immune response could be measured after the *Mh* challenge.
After Mh challenge, most control calves developed severe clinical signs and had to be euthanized on humane grounds. The clinical scores reflected the fatal severity of disease in the controls as opposed to the clearly milder course of the disease in the vaccinated animals. At post mortem examination lung pathology was typical for *Mh*

pneumonia. The lung lesion scores were significantly reduced in the groups vaccinated only with the inactivated vaccine or after concurrent administration by the IN route. The difference between the IM group and the controls was close to significance.
Nasal swab and lung samples from the control calves contained heavier growth of *Mh* than the respective samples from vaccinated groups, while no differences were observed between vaccination with the Mh vaccine alone or simultaneous application of the live IBR marker vaccine
Taken the results regarding the different parameters for vaccine protection together, the simultaneous application of the live IBR marker vaccine did not interfere with the protection afforded by the inactivated BRSV-PI3-Mh combination vaccine.

Marker aspect of inactivated BVD vaccine

Makoschey, B.; Sonnemans, D.; Muñoz Bielsa, J.; Franken, P.; Mars, M.; Santos, L.; Álvarez, M. (2007) Evaluation of the induction of NS3 specific BVDV antibodies using a commercial inactivated BVDV vaccine in immunization and challenge trials. *Vaccine* **25, 6140 - 6145**

In a first study, heifers were vaccinated five times at monthly interval with a commercially available inactivated BVDV vaccine. One group of twelve animals received a double dose at each time point while a second group of six animals was given a single dose at each vaccination. Serum samples taken at monthly interval were tested for NS3 specific antibodies using different commercial BVDV antibody ELISA tests.
At the time of the first and second vaccination, all animals were tested negative in all three BVDV-NS3 antibody tests. After the second vaccination, results varied considerably between the different tests. With the exception of two samples that gave questionable result on study day 90, all samples from animals vaccinated with the single dose regime gave negative results when tested in ELISA-A. In the same test, three and one sample respectively from the group vaccinated with the double dose regime gave a positive result on study days 120 and 150 respectively and only one animal of this group gave a questionable result at day 120. With the two other ELISAs a larger number of samples were tested positive after three or more vaccinations, making these two tests unsuitable as marker test. Interestingly, a lot of animals that were found positive or questionable at one month after the fifth vaccination were tested questionable and negative respectively one month later, indicating that the NS3 antibody response induced by the multiple vaccinations is only of short duration.
The BVDV NS3 specific antibody response after infection of previously vaccinated animals was determined in a second study. Five calves at the age of 3-4 months and seronegative for BVDV were vaccinated with a commercially available inactivated BVDV vaccine according to the standard vaccination schedule. Three weeks after the second vaccination they were inoculated intranasally with a BVDV field isolate. Successful vaccination and infection with BVDV was confirmed by the levels of BVDV-neutralising antibodies.
All animals were tested negative for NS3 specific antibodies until the second vaccination and three out of five animals were still seronegative until one week after challenge. The two other animals had low levels of NS3 specific antibodies at the time of challenge and one week later, as the respective samples gave different results

for the different tests. Most importantly, all animals were found positive in all four ELISA systems from 2 weeks after infection onwards, indicating that the vaccination did not interfere with the NS3 antibody response after infection with BVDV field virus.

Kuijk. H.; Franken, P.; Mars, M.; bij de Weg, W.; Makoschey, B. (2008) Monitoring of a BVDV infection in a vaccinated herd by testing of milk for antibodies against NS3. *The Veterinary Record* 163; 482 - 484

A field study was performed on a Dutch dairy farm to establish, whether the NS3 antibody testing of milk samples (bulk milk or individual milk samples) is suitable for differentiation between BVDV vaccinated and field virus infected animals.

A herd vaccination program for BVDV was initiated in the farm after detection of a PI animal. All animals older than 8 months were vaccinated twice at a four weeks interval with an inactivated BVDV vaccine and vaccinations were repeated every six months. Twelve cows that were seronegative before vaccination and five cows with intermediate neutralizing antibody titers against BVDV before vaccination were selected for further evaluation. Blood samples were taken from these animals immediately prior to each vaccination and four weeks later. At the same time points, individual milk samples and bulk milk samples were collected.

All animals that were seronegative before vaccination developed BVDV neutralizing antibodies after the immunizations. An intercurrent infection with BVDV was diagnosed in three animals as judged by a strong increase in BVDV neutralizing antibody response between vaccinations and neutralizing antibody titers remained at a very high level throughout the observation period.

For the evaluation of the NS3 antibody response, the animals were grouped into three categories: i) animals that were seronegative before vaccination and did not experience a field virus infection (vaccinated / non infected; n=7), ii) animals that were seronegative before vaccination and that were infected after the second dose (vaccinated / infected; n=3) and iii) thirdly, those animals that were already infected before the vaccination was started (infected / vaccinated; n=4).

All samples, serum and milk, from uninfected animals were tested negative for NS3 specific antibodies at all time points. Moreover, all serum samples taken after infection with BVDV virus were tested positive, regardless whether the animals have been vaccinated before or after the infection. Likewise, the overall majority of the milk samples from infected animals were also tested positive in the four NS3 ELISA tests. Those animals that gave a false negative result in a milk sample at a certain sample moment were tested positive again at the next time point. Finally, the bulk milk samples were tested negative on study day 28, but positive in the NS3 ELISA on all other time points indicating that the antibody level at day 28 was close to the detection limit.

Comparing the results obtained in serum with those in milk, both substrates were found appropriate to monitor BVDV infection in a vaccinated herd, even after multiple vaccinations if a suitable NS3 antibody test is used.

Álvarez, M.; Donate, J.; Makoschey, B. Development of antibodies against non-structural proteins of the bovine viral diarrhoea virus in serum and milk samples from vaccinated animals. *Submitted*

Following the design of the previous studies additional studies were performed to compare NS3 antibody levels in milk and serum. Samples were tested using commercially available ELISA tests from different manufacturers. Two separate studies were performed in BVD seronegative herds. In the first study (standard schedule) 48 animals received a basic vaccination of two doses at four weeks interval and were revaccinated 6 months later. Six animals were left unvaccinated. Blood and milk samples were taken at the days of vaccination and four or three weeks later. In the second study (intensive schedule) 20 animals were vaccinated five times at monthly interval with a double dose of the vaccine. A second group of 32 animals received a single dose of the vaccine at the same time points and eight animals served as unvaccinated controls. Serum and milk (individual and bulk) samples were taken at pre-set times. Vaccination according to the standard schedule did not induce antibodies against BVDV NS3 protein with only a few exceptions on serum and milk samples taken three weeks after the third dose. With the intense vaccination schedule antibodies against BVDV NS3 proteins were detected both in serum and milk in different proportions of the animals. After 5 vaccinations with a single dose only 17% of the animals were positive in milk in at least one test and at least one time point. The repeated (5x) application of a double dose induced BVDV NS specific milk antibodies in 60% of the animals, However, three months after the application of the 5th dose all milk samples were tested negative.

The distribution of individual results obtained with the various tests for serum and milk samples from animals vaccinated with the single dose regime according to the intensive schedule followed different patterns. The individual readings on serum samples with two ELISAs varied within a certain range, while results obtained with the two other tests seemed to fall into two distinct categories: The majority of animals gave clearly negative results throughout the study, while only a few animals gave positive results after four or five vaccinations. All three ELISA's applicable for milk testing gave clearly negative results until after five vaccinations for the majority of milk samples.

Another interesting observation was made when results form serum and milk were compared in animals vaccinated with the single dose regime according to the intense schedule. There was no direct correlation between the BVDV NS specific antibody response measured in milk samples and the result of the respective serum sample.

Risk assessment for unintended immunisation of cattle by use of vaccines

Makoschey, B., van Gelder, P.T., Keijsers, V. and Goovaerts, D. (2003) Bovine viral diarrhoea virus antigen in foetal calf serum batches and consequences of such contamination for vaccine production, *Biologicals,* **31, 203-208.**

A study was performed to determine the risk that non-infectious BVDV particles originating from the fetal calf serum (FCS) used during vaccine virus production induce seroconversion against BVDV in cattle. An experimental vaccine was prepared using FCS with a high number of BVDV copies (50% (v/v)) and aluminium hydroxide and aluminium phosphate as adjuvant. Five seronegative calves were inoculated twice at a 4 weeks interval with 4 ml of the vaccine via the intramuscular route. Blood samples were taken at the days of vaccination and two weeks after the second vaccination. All five animals remained seronegative for BVDV-1 and BVDV-2 throughout the entire experiment, indicating that the risk of a seroconversion against BVDV due to inactivated BVDV present in FCS can be neglected.

Makoschey, B. and Beer, M. (2004) Assessment of the risk of transmission of vaccine viruses by using insufficiently cleaned injection devices. *The Veterinary Record,* **155, 563-564**

Re-use of injection devices is common practice in the modern cattle farming. If the devices are insufficiently cleaned after use, remnants of vaccine virus might unintentionally be injected together with another vaccine. As an example it was investigated whether traces of live or inactivated IBR marker vaccines induce seroconversion if administered together with a BVDV vaccine. Six groups of seronegative cattle were vaccinated twice with a commercial inactivated BVDV vaccine. At the first vaccination, the BVDV vaccine was spiked with a live or inactivated IBR marker vaccine at a dilution of 1:50, 1:500 or 1:5000.
Two out of five animals vaccinated with the highest concentration (1:50) of the inactivated IBR marker vaccine developed low levels of BoHV-1 specific antibodies that were detected by BoHV-1 gB antibody ELISA but below the limits of detection in the neutralising antibody test. The three remaining animals in this group and the animals that received lower concentrations of the inactivated IBR marker vaccine remained seronegative for BoHV-1 gB specific antibodies as well as neutralising antibodies.
By contrast, after inoculation of the live IBR marker vaccine, all animals developed specific antibodies regardless of the dilution. Interestingly, the titers of neutralising antibodies were similar for the three virus concentrations used. The levels of immunity in the seropositive animals in this study are probably not sufficient to protect the animals from clinical disease after subsequent infection with BoHV-1 field virus, anyhow the antibody levels would interfere with BoHV-1 monitoring programs.

Makoschey, B. and Beer, M. (2007) A live bovine herpesvirus-1 marker vaccine is not shed after intramuscular vaccination. *Berliner und Münchner Tierärztliche Wochenschrift*, 120, 480-482

It is generally accepted that gE deleted BoHV-1 vaccine viruses are shed with nasal discharge after intranasal vaccination. A study was performed to determine whether animals become viremic and / or excrete vaccine virus with nasal discharge after intramuscular application of the vaccine. Five calves, seronegative for BoHV-1 were vaccinated IM with a high dose of a live IBR marker vaccine.

All animals developed BoHV-1 neutralizing antibodies within 4 weeks after the vaccination, confirming that they have been successfully vaccinated. Nasal swab samples were taken daily for 11 days and all found negative for BoHV-1 virus, demonstrating that the vaccine virus was not shed after IM vaccination. Likewise, none of the animals became viremic as judged by the fact that all blood samples were found negative for BoHV-1 virus and BoHV-1 specific DNA.

These results lead to the recommendation to apply the BoHV-1 marker live vaccine by the IM route in situations where shedding of the vaccine virus should be avoided.

D. Discussion

Critical factors in the development of animal models for the evaluation of vaccine efficacy

Prior to licensing of a veterinary vaccine the safety and efficacy of a vaccine has to be established under controlled conditions (EudraLex 2009). Prevention or reduction of clinical disease is an important criterium for vaccine efficacy. Any label claim with regards to protection against clinical disease has to be supported by study data, which requires suitable disease models. The pathogenesis of a virus is typically studied in animals that are only a few weeks old and do not have maternal immunity. However, for the purpose of vaccine testing disease has to be reproduced in older animals. Moreover, efficacy has to be demonstrated in calves with maternal immunity, if a vaccine is intended for use in this age group. If specific efficacy claims e.g. protection against fetal infection with BVDV, are intended, studies have to be designed accordingly. The demonstration of protection for vaccines that should be marketed in the EU is described in the respective monograph of the European Pharmacopoiea. For vaccines in the USA, the Title 9 of the Code of Federal Regulation (9CFR) applies. In these regulations, a number of parameters, including minimal numbers of animals and time schedules as well as requirements for a valid test are usually well defined, yet they do not provide full protocols as to how the studies have to be performed. Such protocols have to be developed by the vaccine manufacturers. For this purpose, the virulence of potential challenge viruses has to be determined *in vivo* as the genetic basis for the variation in virulence between different virus strains is often unknown. Moreover, the challenge dose and procedure as well as the parameters that allow conclusions regarding protection need to be determined. Here, such studies to develop vaccination-challenge studies for BVDV, BoHV-1 and BRSV are reported. The difficulties to develop suitable protocols for vaccination-challenge studies vary considerably between the three viruses: BoHV-1 and BVDV-2 produced clear signs of clinical disease in unvaccinated control animals, whereas only mild disease was observed after infection with BVDV-1 and BRSV. These results are in general agreement with observations by other groups on the difficulties to reproduce clinical disease after experimental infection with BVDV-1 (Ridpath et al. 2007) and BRSV (Larsen 2000).

Among the animal factors, the status of maternal immunity is probably the most relevant for the successful reproduction of disease. Studies intended for the licensing of veterinary vaccines have to be performed in animals that are representative for the field situation. In the case of BRSV, this means that efficacy has to be demonstrated in the face of MDA. It has been shown, that clinical signs are inversely proportional to the level of passive antibodies (Kimman et al. 1988). Therefore, reproduction of clinical disease after experimental infection of animals with antibodies is deemed to be difficult. However, data obtained from two infection studies with the same challenge virus and following the same protocol demonstrated, that antibody levels are not the only parameter that determines the clinical presentation as the disease was more pronounced in the animals with antibodies (Vangeel et al. 2005). On the other hand, also infection of gnotobiotic calves with BRSV often failed to produce signs of disease (Thomas et al. 1984; Valarcher et al. 2006). The challenge virus and challenge procedure used in the study described here had induced mild to severe respiratory

disease in calves without maternal antibodies (Schmidt et al. 2002), but disease could not be reproduced in calves with passive immunity (**van der Sluijs et al. 2009**).
A related animal factor is the age of the animals. In vaccination-challenge study, animals are typically at least 1-5 months old at the time of infection with the virulent virus. In the infection study with BoHV-1, animals were about 5 weeks of age at the time of challenge infection and developed symptoms of respiratory disease and pyrexia. When the same challenge virus and challenge procedure was applied in calves of this age group, disease was also observed in other studies (Makoschey & Keil 2000b; Makoschey et al. 2002b), but could not consistently be reproduced in animals that were 7 to 8 months old (Patel 2004; Patel et al. 2004). This difference might suggest an age effect on the susceptibility for BoHV-1. On the other hand, others could reproduce typical lesions of IBR in yearling cattle (Bosch et al. 1996). Also in the case of BRSV and BVDV, clinical disease was reported in animals that were challenged during the first weeks of live (Thomas et al. 1984; Ciszewski et al. 1991; Marshall et al. 1996; Liebler-Tenorio et al. 2002; Valarcher et al. 2006), but also in older animals (Marshall et al. 1998; West et al. 1999b; Antonis et al. 2007; Ridpath et al. 2007).
A third animal factor that might determine the outcome of an infection study are breed related differences in the susceptibility for certain diseases, e.g. the Merino breed of sheep are more susceptible for the infection with bluetongue virus (Parsonson 1990). With regards to the three viruses, studied here, Belgian Blue Cattle are known to be more severely affected by respiratory disease due to their lung physiology, however, it is unknown, whether they are also more susceptible for the virus infection.

Besides the animal factors discussed above, the clinical presentation of a virus infection depends on a number of viral factors. First of all, virus strains may vary in virulence. This has been demonstrated by direct comparison of BVDV isolates (Walz et al. 2001; Kelling et al. 2002; Ridpath et al. 2007). Moreover, gE-negative BoHV-1 recombinants generated *in vitro* from several virulent BoHV-1 strains varied in virulence depending on their parent virus (Muylkens et al. 2006). There is evidence that virulent BRSV strains, become attenuated after only a few passages in cell culture. For this reason, numerous BRSV challenge models described in the literature use virus preparations passaged *in vivo* (West et al. 1999a; Antonis et al. 2007; Boxus et al. 2007; Hamers et al. 2007). Disadvantages of this procedure are, i) the risk of contamination with other pathogens, ii) the limited number of challenge doses that can be recovered from one infected animal, and iii) the rather low BRSV virus titer in the challenge inoculum. In the BRSV challenge study reported here, fresh supernatant of a low passage virus was used as inoculum as described elsewhere (Gershwin et al. 1998; Schmidt et al. 2002). In general, this approach results in higher virus titers, as no infectivity gets lost due to freezing and thawing. A disadvantage is that the actual virus titer is unknown at the time of challenge.
The attenuation of BRSV virus isolates during cell culture passages has some practical implications for the testing of genetically engineered mutants. The virus used to prepare the infectious clone is already fairly attenuated after a large number of cell culture passages. Therefore, it is difficult to judge, whether mutations really lead to an apathogenic phenotype (Schmidt et al. 2002). Similarly, the clinical presentation after infection with the recombinant parent of the BVDV mutants with deletions in the 5'-nontranslated region reported herein (Makoschey et al. 2004) was rather mild, making judgements on the attenuation difficult. It has been reported that a virulent BVDV-2 virus was attenuated in cattle after one passage in an elk and 56 passages in different

cell lines of bovine and lapine origin (Deregt et al. 2004). By contrast, inoculation of calves with the BVDV-1 reference strains Oregon C24V and NADL at high dose via multiple routes induced clinical signs of diarrhoea (Polak & Zmudzinski 2000). In the latter study, both viruses used for infection were of the cp biotype. In the studies reported, where heifers were infected with the ncp biotype of the BVDV-2 strain GiI no clinical signs were observed as opposed to the clinical signs of respiratory disease and diarrhoea reported after infection of calves with the cp / ncp pair of GiI (Makoschey et al. 2001). Also other factors might have contributed to this discrepancy, but unpublished results of an earlier study indicated that the pathogenicity of the BVDV-2 challenge strain was related to the cp virus.

The question, whether the virus dose has an effect on the clinical presentation has been clearly demonstrated for the FMD virus (Alexandersen et al. 2002), but is discussed controversially in the case of the BVD virus. Ridpath and colleagues (Ridpath et al. 2007) did not see a dose effect, on the other hand, thrombocytopenia was reported after infection with 10^7 TCID50 of BVDV-2 strain 890, while infection with a ten times lower dose did not affect the platelet counts (Bolin & Ridpath 1992; Walz et al. 2001).

BoHV-1 virus excretion after infection with the virus used in the studies reported here was comparable after infection with 10^6 TCID50 or 10^8 TCID50 but virus excretion was longer after infection with 10^7 TCID50 as compared to the two other doses (Patel et al. 2004; Patel & Shilleto 2005), indicating that there is no dose effect in the titer range used.

In an early infection study with BRSV, virus preparations with titers ranging between 10^5 TCID50 and 10^8 TCID50 have been used, but also the highest dose failed to induce disease in gnotobiotic calves (Thomas et al. 1984). The Snook BRSV strain passaged in calves has been used at a dose of $10^{5.5}$ TCID50 and $10^{7.3}$ TCID50 in two separate studies (Harmeyer et al. 2006; Hamers et al. 2007). Clinical disease was more severe after infection with the lower dose, indicating, that there is no clear dose effect of BRSV, at least not this titer range.

Another factor, that might affect the outcome of an infection study is the route of infection (Alexandersen et al. 2002). In the context of vaccine efficacy testing, the natural route of infection is generally preferred. The intranasal route of infection is generally followed for BoHV-1 to reproduce respiratory disease, but some authors used a nebulizer for this purpose ((Belknap et al. 1999; Van Drunen Littel-Van Den Hurk et al. 2008). Both routes seem to be equally suitable. For practical reasons the intranasal instillation has been used in the BoHV-1 infection studies described herein. Different infection procedures have been described for BRSV: i) intranasal inoculation, ii) intratracheal inoculation, iii) intranasal via aerosol. The latter has been used in the BRSV infection study described herein. Several challenge models apply a combination these procedures (Thomas et al. 1984; Taylor et al. 2005; Letellier et al. 2008), indicating that the route is considered critical for the outcome of the infection, and that the optimal route is unknown.

In most BRSV infection models, the virus is applied on a single day, but Ciszewski and colleagues have induced disease after BRSV inoculation both intranasal and intratracheal for four consecutive days (Ciszewski et al. 1991).

Successful experimental infection with BVDV has been reported both after intranasal and after intravenous inoculation (Corapi et al. 1990; Liebler-Tenorio et al. 2002). It has been demonstrated that vaccination with BVDV-1 provided partial protection against viremia after intravenous inoculation of BVDV-2 (Makoschey et al. 2001). However, it should be noted, that the infection took place shortly after the vaccination, when the level of circulating antibodies were still high. If the infection is done several months after vaccination, protection against intranasal challenge is probably better than against intravenous challenge. The most natural exposure to BVDV is through contact with a PI animal. This approach has been followed by others for fetal infection studies in pregnant cows (Patel et al. 2002; Fulton et al. 2005a; Grooms et al. 2007), but never in acute disease models. A study to determine the efficacy of transmission of BVDV-2 from a PI to naïve in contact animals is reported here (**Makoschey & Janssen 2009**). The transmission was found to be very efficient as all in-contact animals seroconverted within 4 weeks after the first contact with the PI. Therefore, exposure to a persistently infected calf can be considered a suitable method for experimental infection with BVDV-2.

Under field conditions, infection with two or more respiratory pathogens at the same time is very common (Assie et al. 2009), leading to a more severe clinical disease (Babiuk et al. 1988). For enteric pathogens, it has been demonstrated under experimental conditions, that simultaneous infection with two rotaviruses and one coronavirus lead to severe diarrhoea while the single virus preparations caused only mild disease (Makoschey et al. 2009b). This prinicipe might be successful also in the case of BRSV, yet they are currently not accepted by licensing authorities to demonstrate vaccine efficacy. Sequential infection with the individual pathogens has been performed to demonstrate the efficacy of a multivalent vaccine against the individual antigens (Patel 2004) in order to reduce the number of experimental animals. The same approach was followed in the study reported here, to investigate, whether a live IBR marker vaccine has a negative effect on the vaccine efficacy of an inactivated respiratory combination vaccine when both vaccines are applied at the same time (Makoschey et al. 2006).
In the context of BVDV fetal infection studies, dual infection with BVDV-1 and BVDV-2 would only be accepted by the licensing authorities if the control animals are all infected with both species. Two studies described here were performed in pregnant heifers to study the possibility of a dual intranasal infection with BVDV-1 and BVDV-2 to establish fetal infection (**Makoschey & Janssen 2009**). The BVDV-1 and the BVDV-2 strain, were inoculated separately into either nostril result in order to promote fetal infection of the fetus with both viruses. Yet, dual transplacental infection of a fetus with both BVDV species was observed only in one occasion but could not consistently be reproduced. These results are in agreement with earlier studies where inoculation of pregnant heifers with a mixture of two or more BVDV strains resulted in a dual infection of some, but not all fetuses (Brock & Chase 2000; Zimmer et al. 2002). Interestingly, only the BVDV-2 strain established an infection in most of the fetuses in the study reported here, as well as in an earlier study reported by others (Frey et al. 2002). No information is available, whether BVDV-2 has a general competitive advantage over BVDV-1.

In the three infection models described here, different parameters were studied to judge vaccine efficacy. Due to the clear reproducible clinical manifestation of infection with BoHV-1 and the high levels of virus excretion, evaluation of clinical signs, including body temperatures and possibly also weight gain, and quantification of virus levels in nasal discharge are sufficient to determine vaccine efficacy. By contrast, clinical disease is often less pronounced after experimental infection with BVDV and BRSV, as discussed above. Therefore, additional parameters have to be evaluated. In the case of BVDV, counts of white blood cells, lymphocytes and

thrombocytes (especially after infection with BVDV-2) can provide objective information on the severity of the clinical presentation. Macroscopical and histological examination of lesions may also provide important data. However, if necropsy is performed during the acute phase of the disease, this interferes with the attribution of clinical scores.
As clinical signs after experimental infection with BRSV are often rather mild, clinical scores are rarely suitable to judge vaccine efficacy. This problem was also encountered in the BRSV infection study performed to investigate, whether a live IBR marker vaccine has a negative effect on the vaccine efficacy of an inactivated respiratory combination vaccine when both vaccines are applied at the same time (Makoschey et al. 2006). Examination of lung lesions is a common approach to determine the severity of the disease (Schmidt et al. 2002; Taylor et al. 2005; Letellier et al. 2008). This approach of performing a necropsy at pre-set times during the study has the additional advantage that BRSV infection can be determined in different tissues of the respiratory tract and specifically in the lower respiratory tract. These data can be very valuable, as BRSV replication in the upper respiratory tract generally results only in relatively low titers in the nasal discharge. In the study reported here (**van der Sluijs et al. 2009**)) less tissue samples were infected with BRSV in the vaccinated animals as compared to the unvaccinated group.
Given the difficulties to reproduce clinical disease after experimental infection with BRSV, any judgment on vaccine efficacy should also consider results from field studies (Morzaria et al. 1979; Stott et al. 1987; Makoschey et al. 2008).

In conclusion, the difficulties to develop a challenge model differed considerably between the three viruses studied. While infection with BoHV-1 wild type virus reproducibly results in clinical disease and high levels of virus excretion, details such as origin of the challenge virus, virus dose and challenge procedure might be much more critical for BRSV and BVDV. In order to allow conclusions on vaccine efficacy it is essential to evaluate a number of parameters in addition to clinical signs and nasal virus excretion. Attempts to develop a dual (BVDV-1 and BVDV-2) fetal challenge procedure failed. By contrast, the challenge procedure by contact with a PI animal that has been applied by others for BVDV-1 was found to be suitable as challenge procedure also for BVD-2.

Effect of a live infectious bovine rhinotracheitis marker vaccine on the immune response to other cattle vaccines applied at the same time

Live and inactivated IBR marker vaccines are widely applied in control programs in a number of countries of the European Union (Makoschey 2006). Combination of the application of the IBR marker vaccines with vaccinations against other common cattle pathogens is the preferred choice of farmers and veterinarian because they simplify animal handling, and therefore, also reduce costs of vaccination and animal stress. However, without prior demonstration of the safety and efficacy after combined use, no other vaccines may be used within 14 days before or after application of a vaccine. It has been demonstrated that deletion of the gE gene of BoHV-1 leads to the attenuation of the virus (Kaashoek et al. 1994; Muylkens et al. 2006). It is well known that wild type BoHV-1 viruses, modulate the immune response against other pathogens (Bielefeldt & Babiuk 1985), however, the effect of gE deletion mutants of BoHV-1 on immune parameters has not been studied. Studies are described herein that adress the question, whether application of a live IBR marker at the same time as an inactivated BVDV vaccine (Makoschey et al. 2006; Alvarez et al. 2007) or an inactivated combination vaccine against respiratory pathogens (Makoschey et al. 2006) has a negative effect on the efficacy of the inactivated vaccine.

Titers of BVDV specific antibodies were clearly lower when the live IBR marker vaccine was reconstituted in the BVDV vaccine at the first and second dose of the BVD basic vaccination schedule. No such negative effect was seen when the two vaccines were applied at the same time but as separate injections, making an immunosuppressive effect of the IBR marker vaccine unlikely. Moreover, concurrent application of the live IBR marker vaccine did not interfere with the immune response induced by an inactivated respiratory combination vaccine (Makoschey et al. 2006) or an inactivated vaccine against bluetongue (Makoschey et al. 2009c).

The lower antibody response after application of the live IBR marker vaccine at the first and second dose of the BVDV vaccine might be caused by interference. On the other hand, application of the inactivated IBR marker vaccine together with the inactivated BVDV vaccine at the first or second dose did not have an effect on the immune response (Makoschey et al. 2009a). Moreover, inactivated combination vaccines that contain BoHV-1 and BVDV antigens have been developed (Patel 2004; Peters et al. 2004), but the efficacy of the antigens in the combination vaccine was not compared with the respective monovalent vaccines. In unpublished studies with experimental combination vaccines we have observed an interference of a *Leptospira interrogans serovar hardjo* bacterin on the immunogenicity of the inactivated BVDV antigen in the vaccine, while the combined application of an inactivated BVDV vaccine and an inactivated *Leptospira hardjo* vaccine as two separate injections did not have an negative effect on the BVDV specific antibody response (Mawhinney & Makoschey 2008).

Therefore, it remains unclear, why and under which conditions some antigens can interfere with the antibody response against BVDV when applied at the same injection site.

In conclusion, the results indicate that a live IBR marker is not immunosuppressive effect as application of the vaccine at the same time as the first or second dose of the basic vaccination with an inactivated BVDV vaccine or an inactivated combination vaccine against respiratory pathogens had no negative effect on the efficacy of the inactivated vaccines. However, some interference was observed, when the BVDV vaccine was used to reconstitute the live IBR marker vaccine at the first and second dose of the BVDV vaccination schedule.

Evaluation of the marker vaccine concept for an inactivated bovine viral diarrhoea virus vaccine

Control programs for BVDV are ongoing or in preparation in several EU Member States. As for any other control program monitoring of the infection status is a key element in these programs. In the case of BVDV, the objectives for monitoring are i) to identify PI animals, ii) follow the progress of the interventions and iii) to rapidly detect new infections. For obvious reasons, identification of PI animals has to be done on individual animal level. Several diagnostic tests are available to detect an PI animal (Fulton et al. 2006; Hilbe et al. 2007). A diagnostic quick scan consisting of bulk milk tests for virus and antibody, and antibody tests in spot check samples from young stock gives an indication on the herd prevalence as well as the possible

Discussion

presence of a PI (Mars & Van Maanen 2005). Once circulation of BVDV in a herd is stopped, monitoring of antibody levels in the production herd by (bulk) milk testing is the preferred approach for monitoring of new-infections, both because of time and costs. As vaccination against BVDV is required in countries with high cattle density and high prevalence of BVDV, the question was raised, whether the antibody response induced by the vaccines would interfere with the interpretation of serological test results. Most of the commercial BVDV-antibody ELISA tests make use of the NS3 protein as a single protein or in combination with other viral proteins, because it is highly conserved among the pestiviruses (Paton et al. 1991). This very immunogenic protein is produced in the virus replication, both in cell culture and in an infected animal. During the production process of the current inactivated BVDV vaccines a fair proportion of the NS proteins get lost. Therefore it was not surprising when Graham and colleagues reported that some inactivated BVDV vaccines do not induce detectable antibodies against the NS3 proteins (Graham et al. 2003) after a basic vaccination course of two injections at 3 or 4 weeks interval. This observation prompted us to perform further studies to investigate, whether an inactivated BVDV vaccine in combination with a suitable NS3 antibody test has properties of a marker vaccine. This marker approach would have the advantage that introduction of BVDV into a vaccinated herd can be detected much earlier than by serological monitoring of the youngstock tracer population because it takes at least six to nine months before the first PI animal is born after the introduction of BVDV into a herd, and at least another four to six months until seroconversion of the youngstock tracer group is detected. By contrast, circulation of BVDV in the production herd would lead to a seroconversion within two to four weeks.

From a marker vaccine, it is expected that i) animals remain antibody negative even after repeated vaccinations, but ii) also that vaccinated animals seroconvert shortly after infection with field virus. Studies that evaluate these two aspects both for serum and milk samples are described (**Makoschey et al. 2007a**; **Kuijk et al. 2008a**; **Álvarez et al. 2009**). The results of the different studies indicate, that the inactivated BVD vaccine used in here exhibits properties of a marker vaccine when the NS3 antibody levels are measured in a suitable test: after vaccination NS3-specific antibody levels are low or undetectable, but the vaccination did not interfere with the development of antibodies against NS3 after subsequent field virus infection. These conclusions apply both for tests performed on serum samples as well as for milk tests. However, it should be noted, that the vaccine was not originally developed as a marker vaccine. It contains NS proteins owing to the production procedure. Yet NS antigen levels are much lower than the content of protective antigens. This is unlike the marker vaccines, that are based on the absence of marker antigens in the product (van Oirschot et al. 1990; Hulst et al. 1993; Kaashoek et al. 1994). In the studies reported here, vaccination according to the standard schedule did induce serum antibodies against the BVDV NS3 protein in a few animals, while such antibodies were more regularly detected in samples from animals vaccinated according to the intensive schedule. The proportion of positive animals varied between the different tests and depended on the number of vaccinations and the dosing regime. The antibody response was highest at four weeks after the fifth vaccination and declined sharply during the following months. This apparently very short duration of the NS3 specific immune response is remarkable as the immune response against infection with BVDV is generally considered to be long lasting (Fredriksen et al. 1999). After vaccination with the same inactivated BVD vaccine used here, specific virus

neutralising antibodies have been shown to slightly decline with time, but six months after vaccination, titers were still moderate to high (Patel et al. 2002).
In both studies reported here that involved milk testing, antibody levels in milk were lower than in serum. Similar results have been reported elsewhere for one of the ELISAs used in the studies (Kramps et al. 1999), while similar antibody levels were determined in milk and serum using an ELISA that was not applied in the studies reported here (Beaudeau et al. 2001).
The fact that the inactivated BVDV vaccine contains low levels of NS3 proteins has the advantage that he antibody response against the NS proteins after vaccination and challenge infection followed the immunological principles of a booster rather than a primary response. In the cases of marker vaccines, that are based on the absence of marker antigens in the product a strong vaccine-induced immunity may interfere with or delay the detection of field virus infection. Recently the marker concept was described for an inactivated purified bluetongue vaccine in combination with NS antibody tests (Barros et al. 2009). According to those data, vaccinated animals did not consistently develop antibodies against the NS protein, after field virus infection, though the animals did not have a sterile immunity. Therefore, one would expect that a BTV field infection could pass unnoticed in a herd immunized with this vaccine.
Based on the results reported here, it can be concluded that the inactivated BVDV vaccine used in the studies has properties of a marker vaccine, when used in combination with a suitable NS3 specific antibody test. Yet, individual animals may test false-negative or false-positive at individual sampling points. Therefore, the marker concept should only be applied for monitoring of herds, not for diagnostics on individual animal level. Unlike the situation for herpesviruses, where seropositive animals are latently infected carriers of the virus, BVDV seropositive animals have normally cleared the virus and do not infect other animals. Therefore, serological diagnosis on individual animals is not relevant for BVDV epidemiology.
The number of uninfected animals with NS3 antibodies due to the vaccination is considerably lower when the testing is performed prior to the re-vaccination rather than shortly after the re-vaccinations.
All these conclusions apply both for the testing of serum samples as well as for milk samples, but the lower sensitivity of the milk test has to be taken into consideration with regards to the sampling intervals.

Risk assessment for unintended immunisation of cattle by use of vaccines

In a number of BoHV-1 and BVDV control programs absence of antibodies is required to achieve the status "free of BoHV-1" or "free of BVDV" respectively. Detection of such antibodies in one or more animals leads to the loss of this high sanitary status for the whole herd, regardless of the reason for the seroconversion. The loss of the status "free of ..." has an important negative economical impact for the herd. A number of situations related to vaccination procedures which might directly or indirectly lead to the seroconversion of an animal are discussed here.
Firstly, field viruses can be transmitted between herds indirectly by contaminated clothes, instruments or medical products. An example for the suspected transmission of BVD virus from an acutely or persistently BVDV infected calf to another herd with medicinal products used during for dehorning of calves in both herds was reported (Katholm & Houe 2006). In a different study, two out of two calves became infected with BVDV and seroconverted within 21 days after vaccination with a Ringworm

Discussion

vaccine of which the rubber stopper on a vaccine bottle was contaminated with nasal secretions of a PI animal (Niskanen & Lindberg 2003).

Secondly, medical products and particularly vaccines might be contaminated with adventitious agents during the production procedure. Extraneous agents originating from the use of animal derived compounds during cell and/or virus culture have been detected in a number of biological products (**Kreeft et al. 1990; Rabenau et al. 1993; O'Toole et al. 1994; Harasawa & Tomiyama 1994; Harasawa & Sasaki 1995; Senda et al. 1995; Harasawa 1995; Kappeler et al. 1996**). Owing to the biology of the virus and the common usage of bovine fetal serum during vaccine production, BVDV is the most common contaminant. A serious outbreak of BVDV in The Netherlands in 2000 was related to a contaminated live IBR marker vaccine (Falcone et al. 2000). Serum-free production procedures were developed to avoid contamination of vaccines with adventitious viruses (Makoschey et al. 2002b).

The two situations mentioned above have been well studied by others. Both involve infectious wild-type virus and may lead to a disease outbreak. The risk of virus transmission by either of the two situations is particularly high for the BVD virus, not only because of the possibility of persistent infection, but also to fact, that already very low amounts of virus (1 $TCID_{50}$) might cause an infection (Antonis et al. 2004).

Here we describe investigations on the possibilities of an unintended immunization of animals by the use of vaccines. Three different situations that do not involve infectious wild-type virus were assessed:

The risk related to contamination of vaccines with infectious BVDV is well documented. Yet, no information was available whether non-infectious BVDV originating from the fetal calf serum used during vaccine production might induce BVDV specific antibodies after immunization of cattle with the respective product. In the study reported here (Makoschey et al. 2003), it was demonstrated that even an "overdose" of adjuvanted fetal calf serum containing non-infectious BVDV did not induce BVDV specific antibodies when injected into cattle. As the natural host, bovines are the most susceptible species for BVDV. Consequently, these results are also applicable to any other species. In this context, pigs would be the most relevant species as BVDV specific antibodies have been detected in pigs after infection with the virus and shown to interfere with diagnostic tests for the classical swine fever virus (Makoschey et al. 2002a).

The two other scenarios are related to the IBR marker viruses. After vaccination with IBR marker vaccines, cattle become seropositive for BoHV-1 gB but remain seronegative for gE. Incidentally, apparently unvaccinated cattle are found with the same serological status (gB+/gE-) (Mars et al. 2000c). The reasons for this seroconversion to gB remains unclear for the majority of the cases. One of the possible explanations would be the "unnoticed" exposure to gE- IBR marker vaccine viruses. Two different scenarios were evaluated in this respect. Firstly the risk of transmission of vaccine virus (e.g. the IBR marker vaccine virus) by using insufficiently cleaned injection devices was assessed and found to be very high for the live vaccine and still considerable for the inactivated vaccine (Makoschey & Beer 2004). While this unintended "immunization" probably would not elicit a protective immunity, it might interfere with eradication programs and, thus cause serious economic losses.

Another scenario in this context would be transmission of vaccine virus from a vaccinated animal to an unvaccinated in-contact animal. It was well known that gE deleted IBR marker vaccine viruses are excreted with nasal discharge following intranasal vaccination (van Engelenburg et al. 1995; Lemaire et al. 2001) and may be

Discussion

transmitted to in-contact animals, though at a low incidence (Mars et al. 2000a). Attempts to re-activate latent gE- vaccine virus in animals vaccinated intranasally were successful in one study (Lemaire et al. 2001), but not reproduced in another (Mars et al. 2000b). Taken all these information together, the possibility that gE-vaccine virus is transmitted to in-contact animals can not be excluded if the vaccine is applied intranasally. Under practical conditions, the most relevant situation would be virus transmission following re-activation of an animal vaccinated earlier in life. The potential risk associated with virus excretion in the days following intranasal vaccination is less relevant for the field situation, as vaccination should always involve all susceptible animals.

Since no information was available, whether gE deleted BoHV-1 vaccine virus applied intramuscularly establishes a systemic infection, possibly resulting in virus shedding and / or latency, a study described here was performed to answer these questions (Makoschey & Beer 2007). The results demonstrate that the gE-deleted IBR marker vaccine virus does not establish a systemic infection after intramuscular application. Without this information, some users might choose an inactivated vaccine to avoid the risk of vaccine virus shedding. However, a live IBR marker vaccine can offer the advantage of a single dose primary vaccination course (Patel et al. 2004), an early onset of immunity (Makoschey & Keil 2000a) and the possibility to vaccinate animals at a very young age. The findings reported here allow to recommend application of the tested IBR marker live vaccine by the intramuscular route in situations where it is undesirable that the vaccine virus is shed.

In conclusion, the risk of seroconversion against BVDV due to use of FCS batches containing non-infectious BVDV for vaccine production can be neglected. Likewise, cattle vaccinated intramuscularly with a live IBR marker vaccine do not represent a risk for transferring vaccine virus to in-contact animals. By contrast, the risk of unintended transfer of vaccine virus by the use of insufficiently cleaned injection devices was found to be very high, especially for live vaccines.

E. Summary

Vaccines against three economically important cattle viruses, namely BVDV, BoHV-1 and BRSV, were evaluated from different perspectives related to vaccine testing for licensing purposes, but also to different aspects regarding the practical use of vaccines under field conditions.

Challenge models that comply with the relevant regulations are required to demonstrate the efficacy of a vaccine under controlled conditions. Challenge studies and studies performed to develop such models for BoHV-1, BVDV and BRSV are described. The difficulties differed considerably between the three viruses studied. After infection with BoHV-1 wild type, clinical sign and high levels of virus excretion were reproducibly observed. By contrast, disease was less pronounced and virus titers in blood and / or nasal secretions were much lower after infection with BRSV and BVDV. In order to allow conclusions on vaccine efficacy against these two viruses a number of parameters in addition to clinical signs and virus titration should be evaluated. Attempts to develop a dual (BVDV-1 and BVDV-2) fetal challenge procedure failed. By contrast, the challenge procedure by contact with a PI animal that has been applied by others for BVDV-1 was found to be suitable as challenge procedure also for BVD-2.

A very practical question regarding the use of vaccines under field conditions is the possibility to combine vaccination protocols. Separate studies were performed to determine the immune response after combined application of a live IBR marker vaccine and an inactivated BVD vaccine or an inactivated BRSV-PI3-*Mh* vaccine. The results of these studies indicate that a live IBR marker is not immunosuppressive as application of the vaccine at the same time as the first or second dose of the basic vaccination with an inactivated BVDV vaccine or an inactivated combination vaccine against respiratory pathogens had no negative effect on the efficacy of the inactivated vaccines. However, some interference was observed, when the BVDV vaccine was used to reconstitute the live IBR marker vaccine at the first and second dose of the BVDV vaccination schedule.

Different possibilities for interference of vaccination with the interpretation of serological tests in BVDV and IBR disease control programs were investigated. A number of studies were performed to evaluate the question, whether the use of an inactivated BVDV vaccine affects the possibilities to detect a BVDV infection by antibody testing. In this context, both, serum and milk were evaluated as substrate. Based on the results reported here, it was concluded that the inactivated BVDV vaccine used in the studies has properties of a marker vaccine, when used in combination with a suitable NS3 specific antibody test. Yet, this marker concept should only be applied for monitoring of herds, not for diagnostics on individual animal level. Both, serum and milk samples were found suitable as substrates, but the lower sensitivity of the milk test has to be taken into consideration with regards to the sampling intervals.

Further studies were performed to evaluate possible risks of the unintended immunisation by use of vaccines. This question is particularly relevant for BoHV-1 and BVDV as some control programs for these viruses apply monitoring of herds for antibodies to these viruses. The analysis of three different risk situations in this respect led to the following conclusions: Firstly, the risk of seroconversion against BVDV due to use of FCS containing non-infectious BVDV for vaccine production can be neglected. Likewise, cattle vaccinated intramuscularly with a live IBR marker vaccine were found not to represent a risk for transferring vaccine virus to in-contact animals as they did not shed vaccine virus nor did they become viremic. By contrast, the risk of unintended transfer of vaccine virus by the use of insufficiently cleaned injection devices was found to be very high, especially for live vaccines.

The results reported here should be taken into consideration when advice is given on practical use of vaccines against BVDV, BoHV-1 and BRSV.

F. Zusammenfassung

Impfstoffe gegen drei wirtschaftlich bedeutende Virusinfektionen des Rindes, BVDV, BoHV-1 und BRSV, wurden aus unterschiedlichen Perspektiven im Zusammenhang mit der Wirksamkeitsprüfung im Rahmen der Zulassung aber auch unter verschiedenen Aspekten im Bezug auf die praktische Anwendung unter Feldbedingungen untersucht.

Belastungsinfektionsmodelle, welche die Anforderungen der relevanten Richtlinien erfüllen, sind zum Nachweis der Wirksamkeit von Impfstoffen unter kontrollierten Bedingungen erforderlich. Entsprechende Belastungsinfektionen mit BoHV-1, BVDV und BRSV sowie Studien, die zur Entwicklung derartiger Modelle beitragen werden beschrieben. Die Schwierigkeiten variierten stark zwischen den drei untersuchten Viren. So wurden nach Infektion mit BoHV-1 Wildtypvirus wurden deutliche Krankheitssymptome und hochtitrige Virusausscheidung reproduzierbar nachgewiesen. Im Gegensatz dazu waren im Falle von BRSV und BVDV das Krankheitsbild weniger ausgeprägt und die Virustiter im Blut und / oder Nasensekret sehr niedrig. Um Aussagen zur Wirksamkeit von Impfstoffen gegen diese zwei Viren treffen zu können, sollten zusätzlich zum klinischen Bild und dem quantitativen Virusnachweis weitere Parameter untersucht werden. Ansätze zur Entwicklung einer Methode für die gleichzeitige Infektion des Fetus mit BVDV-1 und BVDV-2 waren nicht erfolgreich. Im Gegensatz dazu erwies sich die Methode der Belastungsinfektion durch Kontakt zu einem persistent infizierten Tier, wie sie für BVDV-1 von Anderen bereits angewendet wurde, auch für BVDV-2 als geeignet.

Die Möglichkeit, Impfmassnahmen zu kombinieren ist eine sehr praktische Frage zur Anwendung von Vakzinen im Feld. In verschiedenen Studien wurde die Immunantwort nach gleichzeitiger Applikation einer markierte IBR Lebendvakzine und einer inaktivierten BVD Vakzine oder einer inaktivierten BRSV-PI3-*Mh* Vakzine untersucht. Die Ergebnisse dieser Studien deuten darauf hin, dass die markierte IBR Lebendvakzine nicht imunsuppressiv ist, da nach gleichzeitiger Applikation zusammen mit der ersten oder zweiten Dosis der Basisimpfung mit einer inaktivierten BVD oder einer inaktivierten Vakzine gegen respiratorische Pathogene kein negativer Effekt auf die Wirksamkeit der inaktivierten Impfstoffe festgestellt wurde. Interferenz wurde jedoch festgestellt, wenn sowohl bei der ersten als auch bei der zweiten Dosis der BVD Basisimpfung die inaktivierte BVD Vakzine zur Rekonstituierung der markierten IBR Lebendvakzine verwendet wurde.

Im Folgenden wurden verschiedene Situationen zu einer möglichen Interferenz von Impfmassnahmen mit der Interpretation der serologischen Diagnostik im Rahmen von BVDV und IBR Bekämpfungsprogrammen untersucht. In mehreren Studien wurde der Frage nachgegangen, ob der Einsatz eines inaktivierten BVDV Impfstoffes die Möglichkeit der serologischen Diagnostik zum Nachweis einer BVDV Infektion beeinträchtigt. In diesem Zusammenhang wurden sowohl Serum als auch Milch als Substrat untersucht. Aufgrund der hier beschriebenen Ergebnisse kann gefolgert werden, dass die geprüfte Vakzine Markereigenschaften hat, wenn geeignete NS3 Antikörperteste angewendet werden. Dieses Markerkonzept sollte jedoch nur zur Diagnostik auf Herdenniveau und nicht zur Einzeltierdiagnostik angewendet werden. Sowohl Serum als auch Milch erwiesen sich als geeignet, die geringere Sensitivität der Milchtests sollte jedoch bei der Festlegung der Intervalle für die Probennahme berücksichtigt werden.

Weitere Studien waren erforderlich, um mögliche Risiken einer unbeabsichtigten Immunisierung bei der Anwendung von Impfstoffen zu untersuchen. Diese Frage ist

Zusammenfassung

besonders relevant für BoHV-1 und BVDV, da in einigen Bekämpfungsprogrammen für diese Viren die Überwachung der Herden auf dem Antikörpernachweis beruht. Die Untersuchung von drei verschiedenen Risiken führte zu den folgenden Schlussfolgerungen: Das Risiko einer Serokonversion gegen BVDV durch nicht-infektiöses BVD Virus in fötalem Kälberserum, das zur Impfstoffherstellung verwendet wurde, kann vernachlässigt werden. Ebenso erwies sich, dass Rinder, die intramuskulär mit einer markierten IBR Lebendvakzine geimpft waren kein Risiko für eine Übertragung von Impfvirus auf Kontakttiere darstellen, da sie weder den Impfstoff ausschieden noch virämisch wurden. Im Gegensatz dazu ist das Risiko einer unbeabsichtigten Übertragung von Impfvirus bei der Anwendung unzureichend gereinigter Impfbestecke als sehr hoch zu beurteilen, besonders im Fall von Lebendvakzinen.

Die beschriebenen Ergebnisse sollten bei Empfehlungen zur praktischen Anwendung von Impfstoffen gegen BVDV, BoHV-1 und BRSV berücksichtigt werden.

G. References

Ackermann, M. and Engels, M., 2006. Pro and contra IBR-eradication, *Veterinary Microbiology*, 113, 293-302.

Alexandersen, S., Brotherhood, I. and Donaldson, A.I., 2002. Natural aerosol transmission of foot-and-mouth disease virus to pigs: minimal infectious dose for strain O1 Lausanne, *Epidemiology and Infection*, 128, 301-312.

Alston,J., 2007. BVD Eradication in Norfolk and Suffolk, http://www.rvc.ac.uk/aboutus/staff/jbrownlie/documents/NorfolkSuffolk_Newsletter_apr07.pdf .

Alvarez, M., Bielsa, J.M., Santos, L. and Makoschey, B., 2007. Compatibility of a live infectious bovine rhinotraheitis (IBR) marker vaccine and an inactivated bovine viral diarrhoea virus (BVDV) vaccine, *Vaccine*, 25, 6613-6617.

Álvarez, M., Donate, J. and Makoschey, B., 2009. Development of antibodies against non-structural proteins of the bovine viral diarrhoea virus in serum and milk samples from vaccinated animals, *Submitted*.

Antonis, A.F., Bouma, A., Bree, J.J. and De Jong, M.C., 2004. Comparison of the sensitivity of in vitro and in vivo tests for detection of the presence of a bovine viral diarrhoea virus type 1 strain, *Veterinary Microbiology*, 102, 131-140.

Antonis, A.F., Schrijver, R.S., Daus, F., Steverink, P.J., Stockhofe, N., Hensen, E.J., Langedijk, J.P. and van der Most, R.G., 2003. Vaccine-induced immunopathology during bovine respiratory syncytial virus infection: exploring the parameters of pathogenesis, *Journal of Virology*, 77, 12067-12073.

Antonis, A.F., van der Most, R.G., Suezer, Y., Stockhofe-Zurwieden, N., Daus, F., Sutter, G. and Schrijver, R.S., 2007. Vaccination with recombinant modified vaccinia virus Ankara expressing bovine respiratory syncytial virus (bRSV) proteins protects calves against RSV challenge, *Vaccine*.

Assie, S., Seegers, H., Makoschey, B., Desire-Bousquie, L. and Bareille, N., 2009. Exposure to pathogens and incidence of respiratory disease in young bulls on their arrival at fattening operations in France, *The Veterinary Record*, 165, 195-199.

Babiuk, L.A., Drunen Littel-van den Hurk, S.v. and Tikoo, S.K., 1996. Immunology of bovine herpesvirus 1 infection, *Veterinary Microbiology*, 53, 31-42.

Babiuk, L.A., Lawman, M.J. and Ohmann, H.B., 1988. Viral-bacterial synergistic interaction in respiratory disease, *Advances in Virus Research*, 35, 219-249.

Bachofen, C., Stalder, H., Braun, U., Hilbe, M., Ehrensperger, F. and Peterhans, E., 2008. Co-existence of genetically and antigenically diverse bovine viral diarrhoea viruses in an endemic situation, *Veterinary Microbiology*, 131, 93-102.

Bahnemann, H.G., 1990. Inactivation of viral antigens for vaccine preparation with particular reference to the application of binary ethylenimine, *Vaccine*, 8, 299-303.

References

Barros, S.C., Cruz, B., Luis, T.M., Ramos, F., Fagulha, T., Duarte, M., Henriques, M. and Fevereiro, M., 2009. A DIVA system based on the detection of antibodies to non-structural protein 3 (NS3) of bluetongue virus, *Veterinary Microbiology*, 137, 252-259.

Baule, C., Kulcsar, G., Belak, K., Albert, M., Mittelholzer, C., Soos, T., Kucsera, L. and Belak, S., 2001. Pathogenesis of primary respiratory disease induced by isolates from a new genetic cluster of bovine viral diarrhea virus type I, *Journal of Clinical Microbiology*, 39, 146-153.

Beaudeau, F., Belloc, C., Seegers, H., Assie, S., Sellal, E. and Joly, A., 2001. Evaluation of a blocking ELISA for the detection of bovine viral diarrhoea virus (BVDV) antibodies in serum and milk, *Veterinary Microbiology*, 80, 329-337.

Becher, P., Orlich, M., Kosmidou, A., König, M., Baroth, M. and Thiel, H.J., 1999. Genetic diversity of pestiviruses: identification of novel groups and implications for classification, *Virology*, 262, 64-71.

Becher, P., Orlich, M. and Thiel, H.J., 2001. RNA recombination between persisting pestivirus and a vaccine strain: Generation of cytopathogenic virus and induction of lethal disease, *Journal of Virology*, 75, 6256-6264.

Becher, P., Orlich, M. and Thiel, H.-J., 2000. Mutations in the 5' nontranslated region of bovine viral diarrhea virus result in altered growth characteristics, *Journal of Virology*, 74, 7884-7894.

Becher,P. & Thiel,H.-J. 2002. Genus Pestivirus *(Flaviviridae)*. In: *The Springer Index of Viruses* (Ed. by C.A.Tidona & G.Darai), pp. 327-331. Heidelberg, Germany, Springer-Verlag.

Beck, E. and Strohmaier, K., 1987. Subtyping of European foot-and-mouth disease virus strains by nucleotide sequence determination, *Journal of Virology*, 61, 1621-1629.

Beer, M., Hehnen, H.R., Wolfmeyer, A., Poll, G., Kaaden, O.R. and Wolf, G., 2000. A new inactivated BVDV genotype I and II vaccine. An immunisation and challenge study with BVDV genotype I, *Veterinary Microbiology*, 77, 195-208.

Belknap, E.B., Walters, L.M., Kelling, C., Ayers, V.K., Norris, J., McMillen, J., Hayhow, C., Cochran, M., Reddy, D.N., Wright, J. and Collins, J.K., 1999. Immunogenicity and protective efficacy of a gE, gG and US2 gene-deleted bovine herpesvirus-1 (BHV-1) vaccine, *Vaccine*, 17, 2297-2305.

Bielefeldt, O.H. and Babiuk, L.A., 1985. Viral-bacterial pneumonia in calves: effect of bovine herpesvirus-1 on immunologic functions, *Journal of infectious diseases*, 151, 937-947.

Blackburn, N.K. and Besselaar, T.G., 1991. A study of the effect of chemical inactivants on the epitopes of Rift Valley fever virus glycoproteins using monoclonal antibodies, *Journal of virological methods*, 33, 367-374.

Bolin, S.R., McClurkin, A.W. and Coria, M.F., 1985. Effects of Bovine Viral Diarrhea Virus on the Percentages and Absolute Numbers of Circulating B and T Lymphocytes in Cattle, *American Journal of Veterinary Research*, 46 (4), 884-886.

Bolin, S.R. and Ridpath, J.F., 1992. Differences in virulence between two noncytopathic bovine viral diarrhea viruses in calves, *American Journal of Veterinary Research*, 53, 2157-2163.

Bolin, S.R. and Ridpath, J.F., 1995. Assessment of protection from systemic infection or disease afforded by low to intermediate titres of passively acquired neutralising antibodies against bovine viral diarrhoea virus in calves, *American Journal of Veterinary Research*, 56, 755-759.

Bosch, J.C., de Jong, M.C., Franken, P., Frankena, K., Hage, J.J., Kaashoek, M.J., Maris-Veldhuis, M.A., Noordhuizen, J.P., Van der Poel, W.H., Verhoeff, J., Weerdmeester, K., Zimmer, G.M. and van Oirschot, J.T., 1998. An inactivated gE-negative marker vaccine and an experimental gD-subunit vaccine reduce the incidence of bovine herpesvirus 1 infections in the field, *Vaccine*, 16, 265-271.

Bosch, J.C., Kaashoek, M.J., Kroese, A.H. and van Oirschot, J.T., 1996. An attenuated bovine herpesvirus 1 marker vaccine induces a better protection than two inactivated marker vaccines, *Veterinary Microbiology*, 52, 223-234.

Bouma, A., Elbers, A.R., Dekker, A., de Koeijer, A., Bartels, C., Vellema, P., van der, W.P., van Rooij, E.M., Pluimers, F.H. and De Jong, M.C., 2003. The foot-and-mouth disease epidemic in The Netherlands in 2001, *Preventive Veterinary Medicine*, 57, 155-166.

Boxus, M., Tignon, M., Roels, S., Toussaint, J.F., Walravens, K., Benoit, M.A., Coppe, P., Letesson, J.J., Letellier, C. and Kerkhofs, P., 2007. DNA Immunization with Plasmids Encoding Fusion and Nucleocapsid Proteins of Bovine Respiratory Syncytial Virus Induces a Strong Cell-Mediated Immunity and Protects Calves against Challenge, *Journal of Virology*, 81, 6879-6889.

Brackenbury, L.S., Carr, B.V. and Charleston, B., 2003. Aspects of the innate and adaptive immune responses to acute infections with BVDV, *Veterinary Microbiology*, 96, 337-344.

Brewer, J.M., Conacher, M., Hunter, C.A., Mohrs, M., Brombacher, J. and Alexander, J., 1999. Aluminium hydroxide adjuvant initiates strong antigen-specific Th2 responses in the absence of IL-4 or IL-13-mediated signalling, *Journal of Immunology*, 163, 6448-6454.

Brock, K.V. and Chase, C.C., 2000. Development of a fetal challenge method for the evaluation of bovine viral diarrhea virus vaccines, *Veterinary Microbiology*, 77, 209-214.

Brownlie, J., Clarke, M.C. and Howard, C.J., 1984. Experimental production of fatal mucosal disease in cattle, *The Veterinary Record*, 114, 535-536.

References

Brownlie, J., Clarke, M.C. and Howard, C.J., 1989. Experimental infection of cattle in early pregnancy with a cytopathic strain of bovine virus diarrhoea virus, *Research in Veterinary Science*, 46, 307-311.

Bruderer, U., Swam, H., Haas, B., Visser, N., Brocchi, E., Grazioli, S., Esterhuysen, J.J., Vosloo, W., Forsyth, M., Aggarwal, N., Cox, S., Armstrong, R. and Anderson, J., 2004. Differentiating infection from vaccination in foot-and-mouth-disease: evaluation of an ELISA based on recombinant 3ABC, *Veterinary Microbiology*, 101, 187-197.

Brum, M.C., Coats, C., Sangena, R.B., Doster, A., Jones, C. and Chowdhury, S.I., 2009. Bovine herpesvirus type 1 (BoHV-1) anterograde neuronal transport from trigeminal ganglia to nose and eye requires glycoprotein E, *Journal of Neurovirology*, 15, 196-201.

Brun, A., Albina, E., Barret, T., Chapman, D.A., Czub, M., Dixon, L.K., Keil, G.M., Klonjkowski, B., Le Potier, M.F., Libeau, G., Ortego, J., Richardson, J. and Takamatsu, H.H., 2008. Antigen delivery systems for veterinary vaccine development. Viral-vector based delivery systems, *Vaccine*, 26, 6508-6528.

Bruschke, C.J., Weerdmeester, K., van Oirschot, J.T. and van Rijn, P.A., 1998. Distribution of bovine virus diarrhoea virus in tissues and white blood cells of cattle during acute infection, *Veterinary Microbiology*, 64, 23-32.

Bruschke, C.J.M., Moormann, R.J.M., van Oirschot, J.T. and van Rijn, P.A., 1997. A subunit vaccine based on glycoprotein E2 of bovine viurs diarrhea virus induces fetal protection in sheep against homologous challenge, *Vaccine*, 15, 1940-1045.

Buchholz, U.J., Finke, S. and Conzelmann, K.K., 1999. Generation of bovine respiratory syncytial virus (BRSV) from cDNA: BRSV NS2 is not essential for virus replication in tissue culture, and the human RSV leader region acts as a functional BRSV genome promoter, *Journal of Virology*, 73, 251-259.

Bukreyev, A., Whitehead, S.S., Murphy, B.R. and Collins, P.L., 1997. Recombinant respiratory syncytial virus from which the entire SH gene has been deleted grows efficiently in cell culture and exhibits site-specific attenuation in the respiratory tract of the mouse, *Journal of Virology*, 71, 8973-8982.

Bundesministerium für Ernährung,L.u.V., 2008. Verordnung zum Schutz der Rinder vor einer Infektion mit dem Bovinen-Virusdiarrhoe-Virus (BVDV-Verordnung, Bundesgesetzblatt Jahrgang 2008 Teil I Nr.59 , 2461.

Burgin, L., Gloster, J. and Mellor, P.S., 2009. Why were there no outbreaks of bluetongue in the UK during 2008?, *The Veterinary Record*, 164, 384-387.

C.F.R., 2009. Title 9 (Animals and Animal Products) Code of Federal Regulations, http://ecfr. gpoaccess. gov/cgi/t/text/text-idx?c=ecfr&tpl=/ecfrbrowse/Title09/9cfr2_main_02. tpl.

Campadelli-Fiume, G., Cocchi, F., Menotti, L. and Lopez, M., 2000. The novel receptors that mediate the entry of herpes simplex viruses and animal alphaherpesviruses into cells, *Reviews in medical virology*, 10, 305-319.

References

Cannon, M.J., Openshaw, P.J. and Askonas, B.A., 1988. Cytotoxic T cells clear virus but augment lung pathology in mice infected with respiratory syncytial virus, *Journal of Experimental Medicine*, 168, 1163-1168.

Carlsson, U., Fredriksson, G., Alenius, S. and Kindahl, H., 1989. Bovine virus diarrhoea virus, a cause of early pregnancy failure in the cow, *Zentralblatt Veterinärmedizin A*, 36, 15-23.

Carman, S., van Dreumel, T., Ridpath, J.F., Hazlett, M., Alves, D., Dubovi, E., Tremblay, R., Bolin, S.R., Godkin, A. and Anderson, N., 1998. Severe acute bovine viral diarrhea in Ontario, 1993-1995, *Journal of Veterinary Diagnostic Investigation*, 10, 27-35.

CD 64/432/EEC, 1964. Article 10 Council Directive 64/432/EEC of 26 June 1964 on animal health problems affecting intra-Community trade in bovine animals and swine, *Eur-Lex 31964L0432*.

CD 91/412/EEC, 1991. Commission Directive 91/412/EEC of 23 July 1991 laying down the principles and guidelines of good manufacturing practice for veterinary medicinal products, *Official Journal L 228* 70-73.

Charleston, B., Brackenbury, L.S., Carr, B.V., Fray, M.D., Hope, J.C., Howard, C.J. and Morrison, W.I., 2002. Alpha/beta and gamma interferons are induced by infection with noncytopathic bovine viral diarrhea virus in vivo, *Journal of Virology*, 76, 923-927.

Charleston, B., Fray, M.D., Baigent, S., Carr, B.V. and Morrison, W.I., 2001. Establishment of persistent infection with non-cytopathic bovine viral diarrhoea virus in cattle is associated with a failure to induce type I interferon, *Journal of General Virology*, 82, 1893-1897.

Cherrie, A.H., Anderson, K., Wertz, G.W. and Openshaw, P.J., 1992. Human cytotoxic T cells stimulated by antigen on dendritic cells recognize the N, SH, F, M, 22K, and 1b proteins of respiratory syncytial virus, *Journal of Virology*, 66, 2102-2110.

Ciszewski, D.K., Baker, J.C., Slocombe, R.F., Reindel, J.F., Haines, D.M. and Clark, E.G., 1991. Experimental reproduction of respiratory tract disease with bovine respiratory syncytial virus, *Veterinary Microbiology*, 28, 39-60.

Collen, T., Carr, V., Parsons, K., Charleston, B. and Morrison, W.I., 2002. Analysis of the repertoire of cattle CD4(+) T cells reactive with bovine viral diarrhoea virus, *Veterinary Immunology and Immunopathology*, 87, 235-238.

Collen, T. and Morrison, W.I., 2000. CD4(+) T-cell responses to bovine viral diarrhoea virus in cattle, *Virus Research*, 67, 67-80.

Collins, J.R., Teegarden, R.M., MacVean, D.W., Smith, G.H., Frank, G.R. and Salman, 1988. Prevalence and specificity of antibodies to bovine respiratory syncytial virus in sera from feedlot and range cattle, *American Journal of Veterinary Research*, 49, 1316-1319.

References

Collins, M.E., Heaney, J., Thomas, C.J. and Brownlie, J., 2009. Infectivity of pestivirus following persistence of acute infection, *Veterinary Microbiology*, 138, 289-296.

Collins,P.L., Chanock,R.M. & Murphy,B.R. 2001. Respiratory syncytial virus. In: *Fields Virology* (Ed. by D.M.Knipe & P.M.Howley), pp. 1443-1485. Philadelphia, Lippincott Williams and Wilkins.

Conceicao, M.M., Tonso, A., Freitas, C.B. and Pereira, C.A., 2007. Viral antigen production in cell cultures on microcarriers Bovine parainfluenza 3 virus and MDBK cells, *Vaccine*, 25, 7785-7795.

Conraths, F.J., Gethmann, J.M., Staubach, C., Mettenleiter, T.C., Beer, M. and Hoffmann, B., 2009. Epidemiology of bluetongue virus serotype 8, Germany, *Emergerging infectious diseases*, 15, 433-435.

Corapi, W.V., Elliott, R.D., French, T.W., Arthur, D.G., Bezek, D.M. and Dubovi, E., 1990. Thrombocytopenia and hemorrhages in veal calves infected with bovine viral diarrhea virus, *Journal of American Veterinary Medicine Association*, 196, 590-596.

Coria, M.F. and McClurkin, A.W., 1978. Duration of active and colostrum-derived passive antibodies to bovine viral diarrhea virus in calves, *Canadian Journal of Comparative Medicine*, 42, 239-243.

Del Medico Zajac, M.P., Puntel, M.Z.P.I., Sadir, A.M. and Romera, S.A., 2006. BHV-1 vaccine induces cross-protection against BHV-5 disease in cattle, *Research in Veterinary Science*, XX, XX.

Dercksen, D., Groot, N.N., Paauwe, R., Backx, A., van Rijn, P. and Vellema, P., 2007. [First outbreak of bluetongue in goats in The Netherlands], *Tijdschrift voor Diergeneeskunde*, 132, 786-790.

Deregt, D., Jacobs, R.M., Carman, P.S. and Tessaro, S.V., 2004. Attenuation of a virulent type 2 bovine viral diarrhea virus, *Veterinary Microbiology*, 100, 151-161.

Dispas, M., Schynts, F., Lemaire, M., Letellier, C., Vanopdenbosch, E., Thiry, E. and Kerkhofs, P., 2003. Isolation of a glycoprotein E-deleted bovine herpesvirus type 1 strain in the field, *The Veterinary Record*, 153, 209-212.

Donis, R.O., Corapi, W. and Dubovi, E.J., 1988. Neutralizing monoclonal antibodies to bovine viral diarrhoea virus bind to the 56K to 58K glycoprotein, *Journal of General Virology*, 69 (Pt 1), 77-86.

Dupuis, L., Deville, S., Aucouturier, J., Ascarateil, S., Laval, A. and Ganne, V., 2009. Veterinary vaccine adjuvants, *Veterinary Immunology and Immunopathology*, 128, 248-249.

Durbin, J.E. and Durbin, R.K., 2004. Respiratory syncytial virus-induced immunoprotection and immunopathology, *Viral Immunology*, 17, 370-380.

Elahi, S.M., Shen, S.H., Talbot, B.G., Massie, B., Harpin, S. and Elazhary, Y., 1999a. Induction of humoral and cellular immune responses against the nucleocapsid of bovine viral diarrhea virus by an adenovirus vector with an inducible promoter, *Virology*, 261, 1-7.

Elahi, S.M., Shen, S.H., Talbot, B.G., Massie, B., Harpin, S. and Elazhary, Y., 1999b. Recombinant adenoviruses expressing the E2 protein of bovine viral diarrhea virus induce humoral and cellular immune responses, *FEMS Microbiological Letters*, 177, 159-166.

Ellis, J.A., Hassard, L.E., Cortese, V.S. and Morley, P.S., 1996a. Effects of perinatal vaccination on humoral and cellular immune responses in cows and young calves [see comments], *Journal of the American Veterinary Medical Association*, 208, 393-400.

Ellis, J.A., Philibert, H., West, K., Clark, E., Martin, K. and Haines, D., 1996b. Fatal pneumonia in adult dairy cattle associated with active infection with bovine respiratory syncytial virus, *Canadian Veterinary Journal*, 37, 103-105.

Ellis, J.A., West, K.H., Waldner, C. and Rhodes, C., 2005. Efficacy of a saponin-adjuvanted inactivated respiratory syncytial virus vaccine in calves, *Canadian Veterinary Journal*, 46, 155-162.

Elvander, M., 1996. Severe respiratory disease in dairy cows caused by infection with bovine respiratory syncytial virus, *The Veterinary Record*, 138, 101-105.

Endsley, J.J., Roth, J.A., Ridpath, J. and Neill, J., 2003. Maternal antibody blocks humoral but not T cell responses to BVDV, *Biologicals*, 31, 123-125.

Engels, M. and Ackermann, M., 1996. Pathogenesis of ruminant herpesvirus infections, *Veterinary Microbiology*, 53, 3-15.

Engels, M., Palatini, M., Metzler, A.E., Probst, U., Kihm, U. and Ackermann, M., 1992. Interactions of bovine and caprine herpesviruses with the natural and the foreign hosts, *Veterinary Microbiology*, 33, 69-78.

EudraLex, 2009. EudraLex - Volume 5 - Pharmaceutical Legislation Medicinal Products for veterinary use, http://ec.europa.eu/enterprise/pharmaceuticals/eudralex/vol5_en.htm .

European Thematic Network on Bovine Viral Diarrhoea Virus (BVDV), 2001. Position Paper BVDV Control in Europe, *http://www. bvdv-contro. org*.

Ezanno, P., Fourichon, C., Viet, A.F. and Seegers, H., 2007. Sensitivity analysis to identify key-parameters in modelling the spread of bovine viral diarrhoea virus in a dairy herd, *Preventive Veterinary Medicine*, 80, 49-64.

Falcone, E., Tollis, M. and Conti, G., 2000. Bovine Viral Diarrea disease associated with contaminated vaccine, *Vaccine*, 18, 387-388.

Ferrer, F., Zoth, S.C., Calamante, G. and Taboga, O., 2007. Induction of virus-neutralizing antibodies by immunization with Rachiplusia nu per os infected with a recombinant baculovirus expressing the E2 glycoprotein of bovine viral diarrhea virus, *Journal of Virological Methods*, 146, 424-427.

Fogg, M.H., Parsons, K.R., Thomas, L.H. and Taylor, G., 2001. Identification of CD4+ T cell epitopes on the fusion (F) and attachment (G) proteins of bovine respiratory syncytial virus (BRSV), *Vaccine*, 19, 3226-3240.

Fray, M.D., Mann, G.E., Clarke, M.C. and Charleston, B., 2000. Bovine viral diarrhoea virus: its effects on ovarian function in the cow, *Veterinary Microbiology*, 77, 185-194.

Fredriksen, B., Sandvik, T., Loken, T. and Odegaard, S.A., 1999. Level and duration of serum antibodies in cattle infected experimentally and naturally with bovine virus diarrhoea virus, *The Veterinary Record*, 144, 111-114.

Frey, H.R., Eicken, K., Grummer, B., Kenklies, S., Oguzoglu, T.C. and Moennig, V., 2002. Foetal protection against bovine virus diarrhoea virus after two-step vaccination, *Journal of Veterinary Medicine B*, 49, 489-493.

Fritzemeier, J., Haas, L., Liebler, E., Moennig, V. and Greiser-Wilke, I., 1997. The development of early vs. late onset mucosal disease is a consequence of two different pathogenic mechanisms, *Archives of Virology*, 142, 1335-1350.

Fulton, R.W., Briggs, R.E., Ridpath, J.F., Saliki, J.T., Confer, A.W., Payton, M.E., Duff, G.C., Step, D.L. and Walker, D.A., 2005a. Transmission of bovine viral diarrhea virus 1b to susceptible and vaccinated calves by exposure to persistently infected calves, *Canadian Journal of Veterinary Research*, 69, 161-169.

Fulton, R.W., Hessman, B., Johnson, B.J., Ridpath, J.F., Saliki, J.T., Burge, L.J., Sjeklocha, D., Confer, A.W., Funk, R.A. and Payton, M.E., 2006. Evaluation of diagnostic tests used for detection of bovine viral diarrhea virus and prevalence of subtypes 1a, 1b, and 2a in persistently infected cattle entering a feedlot, *Journal of American Veterinary Medicine Association*, 228, 578-584.

Fulton, R.W., Ridpath, J.F., Ore, S., Confer, A.W., Saliki, J.T., Burge, L.J. and Payton, M.E., 2005b. Bovine viral diarrhoea virus (BVDV) subgenotypes in diagnostic laboratory accessions: distribution of BVDV1a, 1b, and 2a subgenotypes, *Veterinary Microbiology*, 111, 35-40.

Gallegos, R.M.G., Larios, E.L.E., Ramirez, L.R., Schmid, R.K. and Aguilar-Setien, A., 1995. Rabies veterinary virus vaccine produced in BHK-21 cells grown on microcarriers a bioreactor, *Archives of Medical Research*, 26, 59-63.

Gerdts, V., Beyer, J., Lomniczi, B. and Mettenleiter, T.C., 2000. Pseudorabies virus expressing bovine herpesvirus 1 glycoprotein B exhibits altered neurotropism and increased neurovirulence, *Journal of Virology*, 74, 817-827.

Gershwin, L.J., Schelegle, E.S., Gunther, R.A., Anderson, M.L., Woolums, A.R., LaRochelle, D.R., Boyle, G.A., Friebertshauser, K.E. and Singer, R.S., 1998. A bovine model of vaccine enhanced respiratory syncytial virus pathophysiology, *Vaccine*, 16, 1225-1236.

Glenny, A.T., Buttle, G.A.H. and Stevens, M.F., 1931. Rate of disappearance of diphtheria toxoid injected into rabbits and guinea-pigs: toxoid precipitated with alum, *Journal of Pathology*, 34, 267-275.

References

Glenny, A.T., Pope, C.G., Waddington, H. and Wallace, U., 1926. Immunological notes XVII to XXIV, *Journal of Pathology*, 29, 31-40.

Glew, E.J. and Howard, C.J., 2001. Antigen-presenting cells from calves persistently infected with bovine viral diarrhoea virus, a member of the Flaviviridae, are not compromised in their ability to present viral antigen, *Journal of General Virology*, 82, 1677-1685.

Graham, D.A., German, A., Mawhinney, K.A. and Goodall, E.A., 2003. Antibody responses of naive cattle to two inactivated bovine viral diarrhoea virus vaccines, measured by indirect and blocking ELISA's and virus neutralisation, *The Veterinary Record*, 152, 795-800.

Grooms, D.L., Bolin, S.R., Coe, P.H., Borges, R.J. and Coutu, C.E., 2007. Fetal protection against continual exposure to bovine viral diarrhea virus following administration of a vaccine containing an inactivated bovine viral diarrhea virus fraction to cattle, *American Journal of Veterinary Research*, 68, 1417-1422.

Grummer, B., Beer, M., Liebler-Tenorio, E. and Greiser-Wilke, I., 2001. Localization of viral proteins in cells infected with bovine viral diarrhoea virus, *Journal of General Virology*, 82, 2597-2605.

Grummer, B., Bendfeldt, S., Wagner, B. and Greiser-Wilke, I., 2002. Induction of the intrinsic apoptotic pathway in cells infected with cytopathic bovine virus diarrhoea virus, *Virus Research*, 90, 143-153.

Hage, J.J., Glas, R.D., Westra, H.H., Maris-Veldhuis, M.A., van Oirschot, J.T. and Rijsewijk, F.A., 1998. Reactivation of latent bovine herpesvirus 1 in cattle seronegative to glycoproteins gB and gE, *Veterinary Microbiology*, 60, 87-98.

Hägglund, S., Svensson, C., Emanuelson, U., Valarcher, J.F. and Alenius, S., 2006. Dynamics of virus infections involved in the bovine respiratory disease complex in Swedish dairy herds, *The Veterinary Journal*, 172, 320-328.

Hall, C.B., Walsh, E.E., Long, C.E. and Schnabel, K.C., 1991. Immunity to and frequency of reinfection with respiratory syncytial virus, *Journal of Infectious Diseases*, 163, 693-698.

Hamers, C., Dehan, P., Couvreur, B., Letellier, C., Kerkhofs, P. and Pastoret, P.P., 2001. Diversity among bovine pestiviruses, *Veterinary Journal*, 161, 112-122.

Hamers, C., di Valentin, E., Lecomte, C., Lambot, M., Joris, E., Genicot, B. and Pastoret, P.P., 2000. Virus neutralizing antibodies against a panel of 18 BVDV isolates in calves vaccinated with Rispoval RS-BVD, *Journal of Veterinary Medicine B*, 47, 721-726.

Hamers, C., Juillard, V. and Fischer, L., 2007. DNA vaccination against pseudorabies virus and bovine respiratory syncytial virus infections of young animals in the face of maternally derived immunity, *Journal of Comparative Pathology*, 137 Suppl 1, S35-S41.

Harasawa, R., 1995. Adventitious pestivirus RNA in live virus vaccines against bovine and swine diseases, *Vaccine*, 13, 100-103.

Harasawa, R. and Sasaki, T., 1995. Sequence analysis of the 5' untranslated region of pestivirus RNA demonstrated in interferons for human use, *Biologicals*, 23, 263-269.

Harasawa, R. and Tomiyama, T., 1994. Evidence of pestivirus RNA in human virus vaccines, *Journal of Clinical Microbiology*, 32, 1604-1605.

Harmeyer, S.S., Murray, J., Imrie, C., Wiseman, A. and Salt, J.S., 2006. Efficacy of a live bovine respiratory syncytial virus vaccine in seropositive calves, *The Veterinary Record*, 159, 456-457.

Harpin, S., Hurley, D.J., Mbikay, M., Talbot, B. and Elazhary, Y., 1999. Vaccination of cattle with a DNA plasmid encoding the bovine viral diarrhoea virus major glycoprotein E2, *Journal of General Virology*, 80, 3137-3144.

Herbert W.J., 1968. The mode of action of mineral oil emulsion adjuvants on antibody production, *Immunology*, 14, 301-318.

Hilbe, M., Stalder, H., Peterhans, E., Haessig, M., Nussbaumer, M., Egli, C., Schelp, C., Zlinszky, K. and Ehrensperger, F., 2007. Comparison of five diagnostic methods for detecting bovine viral diarrhea virus infection in calves, *Journal of Veterinary Diagnostic Investigation*, 19, 28-34.

Howard, C.J., Clarke, M.C. and Brownlie, J., 1989. Protection against respiratory infection with bovine virus diarrhoea virus by passively acquired antibody, *Veterinary Microbiology*, 19, 195-203.

Hulst, M.M., Westra, D.F., Wensvoort, G. and Moormann, R.J., 1993. Glycoprotein E1 of hog cholera virus expressed in insect cells protects swine from hog cholera, *Journal of Virology*, 67, 5435-5442.

Hurtado, A., Garcia-Perez, A.L., Aduriz, G. and Juste, R.A., 2003. Genetic diversity of ruminant pestiviruses from Spain, *Virus Research*, 92, 67-73.

Hutchings, D.L., Campos, M., Qualtiere, L. and Babiuk, L.A., 1990a. Inhibition of antigen-induced and interleukin-2-induced proliferation of bovine peripheral blood leukocytes by inactivated bovine herpes virus 1, *Journal of Virology*, 64, 4146-4151.

Hutchings, D.L., Van Drunen Littel-Van Den Hurk and Babiuk, L.A., 1990b. Lymphocyte proliferative responses to separated bovine herpesvirus 1 proteins in immune cattle, *Journal of Virology*, 64, 5114-5122.

Jansen, T., Hofmans, M.P.M., Theelen, M.J.G., Manders, F. and Schijns, V.E.J.C., 2006. Structure- and oil type-based efficacy of emulsion adjuvants, *Vaccine*, 24, 5400-5405.

Johnson, T.R. and Graham, B.S., 1999. Secreted respiratory syncytial virus G glycoprotein induces interleukin-5 (IL-5), IL-13, and eosinophilia by an IL-4-independent mechanism, *Journal of Virology*, 73, 8485-8495.

References

Joly, A., Fourichon, C. and Beaudeau, F., 2005. Description and first results of a BVDV control scheme in Brittany (western France), *Preventive Veterinary Medicine*, 72, 209-213.

Kaashoek, M.J., Moerman, A., Madic, J., Rijsewijk, F.A., Quak, J., Gielkens, A.L. and van Oirschot, J.T., 1994. A conventionally attenuated glycoprotein E-negative strain of bovine herpesvirus type 1 is an efficacious and safe vaccine, *Vaccine*, 12, 439-444.

Kaashoek, M.J., Rijsewijk, F.A., Ruuls, R.C., Keil, G.M., Thiry, E., Pastoret, P.P. and van Oirschot, J.T., 1998. Virulence, immunogenicity and reactivation of bovine herpesvirus 1 mutants with a deletion in the gC, gG, gI, gE, or in both the gI and gE gene, *Vaccine*, 16, 802-809.

Kaashoek, M.J., Rijsewijk, F.A. and van Oirschot, J.T., 1996. Persistence of antibodies against bovine herpesvirus 1 and virus reactivation two to three years after infection, *Veterinary Microbiology*, 53, 103-110.

Kahn, J.S., Schnell, M.J., Buonocore, L. and Rose, J.K., 1999. Recombinant vesicular stomatitis virus expressing respiratory syncytial virus (RSV) glycoproteins: RSV fusion protein can mediate infection and cell fusion, *Virology*, 254, 81-91.

Kahrs, R.F. 2001. Infectious Bovine Rhinotracheitis and Infectious Pustular Vulvovaginitis. In: *Viral Diseases of Cattle*, pp. 159-170. Iowa State University Press Ames.

Kahrs, R.F. and Smith, R.S., 1965. Infectious bovine rhinotracheitis, infectious pustular vulvovaginitis and abortion in a New York dairy herd, *Journal of the American Veterinary Medical Association*, 146, 217-220.

Kampa, J., Stahl, K., Renstrom, L.H. and Alenius, S., 2007. Evaluation of a commercial Erns-capture ELISA for detection of BVDV in routine diagnostic cattle serum samples, *Acta Veterinaria Scandinavia*, 49, 7.

Kampa, J., Alenius, S., Emanuelson, U., Chanlun, A. and Aiumlamai, S., 2009. Bovine herpesvirus type 1 (BHV-1) and bovine viral diarrhoea virus (BVDV) infections in dairy herds: Self clearance and the detection of seroconversions against a new atypical pestivirus, *The Veterinary Journal*, 182, 223-230.

Kapikian, A.Z., Mitchell, R.H., Chanock, R.M., Shvedoff, R.A. and Stewart, C.E., 1969. An epidemiologic study of altered clinical reactivity to respiratory syncytial (RS) virus infection in children previously vaccinated with an inactivated RS virus vaccine, *American Journal of Epidemiology*, 89, 405-421.

Kappeler, A., Lutz-Wallace, C., Sapp, T. and Sidhu, M., 1996. Detection of bovine polyomavirus contamination in fetal bovine sera and modified live viral vaccines using polymerase chain reaction, *Biologicals*, 24, 131-135.

Karger, A., Schmidt, U. and Buchholz, U.J., 2001. Recombinant bovine respiratory syncytial virus with deletions of the G or SH genes: G and F proteins bind heparin, *Journal of General Virology*, 82, 631-640.

References

Katholm, J. and Houe, H., 2006. Possible spread of bovine viral diarrhoea virus by contaminated medicine, *The Veterinary Record*, 158, 798-799.

Kelling, C.L., Steffen, D.J., Topliff, C.L., Eskridge, K.M., Donis, R.O. and Higuchi, D.S., 2002. Comparative virulence of isolates of bovine viral diarrhea virus type II in experimentally inoculated six- to nine-month-old calves, *American Journal of Veterinary Research*, 63, 1379-1384.

Kendric, J.W., York, C.J. and McKercher, D.G., 1956. A controlled field trial of a vaccine for infectious bovine rhinotracheitis, *Proceedings of the US Livestock Sanitary Association*, 60, 155-158.

Kerkhofs, P., Renjifo, X., Toussaint, J.F., Letellier, C., Vanopdenbosch, E. and Wellemans, G., 2003. Enhancement of the immune response and virological protection of calves against bovine herpesvirus type 1 with an inactivated gE-deleted vaccine, *The Veterinary Record*, 152, 681-686.

Kim, H.W., Canchola, J.G., Brandt, C.D., Pyles, G., Chanock, R.M., Jensen, K. and Parrott, R.H., 1969. Respiratory syncytial virus disease in infants despite prior administration of antigenic inactivated vaccine, *American Journal of Epidemiology*, 89, 422-434.

Kimman, T.G., Sol, J., Westenbrink, F. and Straver, P.J., 1989. A severe outbreak of respiratory tract disease associated with bovine respiratory syncytial virus probably enhanced by vaccination with modified live vaccine, *The Veterinary Quarterly*, 11, 250-253.

Kimman, T.G., Westenbrink, F., Schreuder, B.E. and Straver, P.J., 1987. Local and systemic antibody response to bovine respiratory syncytial virus infection and reinfection in calves with and without maternal antibodies, *Jounal of Clinical Microbiology*, 25, 1097-1106.

Kimman, T.G., Zimmer, G.M., Westenbrink, F., Mars, J. and van Leeuwen, E., 1988. Epidemiological study of bovine respiratory syncytial virus infections in calves: influence of maternal antibodies on the outcome of disease, *The Veterinary Record*, 123, 104-109.

König, P., Beer, M., Makoschey, B., Teifke, J.P., Polster, U., Giesow, K. and Keil, G.M., 2003. Recombinant virus-expressed bovine cytokines do not improve efficacy of a bovine herpesvirus 1 marker vaccine strain, *Vaccine*, 22, 202-212.

Kramps, J.A., Van Maanen, C., van de, W.G., Stienstra, G., Quak, S., Brinkhof, J., Ronsholt, L. and Nylin, B., 1999. A simple, rapid and reliable enzyme-linked immunosorbent assay for the detection of bovine virus diarrhoea virus (BVDV) specific antibodies in cattle serum, plasma and bulk milk, *Veterinary Microbiology*, 64, 135-144.

Kreeft, H.A.J.G., Greiser-Wilke, I., Moennig, V. and Horzinek, M.C., 1990. Attempts to characterize bovine viral diarrhoe virus isolated from cattle after immunization with a contaminated vaccine, *Deutsche Tierärztliche Wochenschrift*, 97, 63-65.

Krempl, C., Murphy, B.R. and Collins, P.L., 2002. Recombinant respiratory syncytial virus with the G and F genes shifted to the promoter-proximal positions, *Journal of Virology*, 76, 11931-11942.

Kuhn, R.J., Griffin, D.E., Zhang, H., Niesters, H.G. and Strauss, J.H., 1992. Attenuation of Sindbis virus neurovirulence by using defined mutations in nontranslated regions of the genome RNA, *Journal of Virology*, 66, 7121-7127.

Kuijk, H., Franken, P., Mars, M.H., de Weg, W.B. and Makoschey, B., 2008a. Monitoring of BVDV in a vaccinated herd by testing milk for antibodies to NS3 protein, *The Veterinary Record*, 163, 482-484.

Kuijk, H., Jansen, M., Moulin, V. and Makoschey, B., 2008b. [Vaccination against bluetongue serotype 8 in the Netherlands], *Tijdschrift voor Diergeneeskunde*, 133, 1006-1009.

Lambot, M., Douart, A., Joris, E., Letesson, J.J. and Pastoret, P.P., 1997. Characterization of the immune response of cattle against non-cytopathic and cytopathic biotypes of bovine viral diarrhoea virus, *Journal of General Virology*, 78, 1041-1047.

Larsen, L.E., 2000. Bovine respiratory syncytial virus (BRSV): a review, *Acta Veterinaria Scandinavia*, 41, 1-24.

Larsen, L.E., Tegtmeier, C. and Pedersen, E., 2001. Bovine respiratory syncytial virus (BRSV) pneumonia in beef calf herds despite vaccination, *Acta Veterinaria Scandinavia*, 42, 113-121.

Lekeux, P., Amory, H., Desmecht, D., Gustin, P., Linden, A. and Rollin, F., 1994. Oxygen transport chain in double-muscled blue Belgian cattle, *British Veterinary Journal*, 150, 463-471.

Lemaire, M., Meyer, G., Baranowski, E., Schynts, F., Wellemans, G., Kerkhofs, P. and Thiry, E., 2000a. Production of bovine herpesvirus type 1-seronegative latent carriers by administration of a live-attenuated vaccine in passively immunized calves, *Journal of Clinical Microbiology*, 38, 4233-4238.

Lemaire, M., Schynts, F., Meyer, G., Georgin, J., Baranowski, E., Gabriel, A., Ros, C., Belak, S. and Thiry, E., 2001. Latency and reactivation of a glycoprotein E negative bovine herpesvirus type 1 vaccine: influence of virus load and effect of specific maternal antibodies, *Vaccine*, 19, 4795-4804.

Lemaire, M., Weynants, V., Godfroid, J., Schynts, F., Meyer, G., Letesson, J.J. and Thiry, E., 2000b. Effects of bovine herpesvirus type 1 infection in calves with maternal antibodies on immune response and virus latency, *Journal of Clinical Microbiology*, 38, 1885-1894.

Letellier, C., Boxus, M., Rosar, L., Toussaint, J.F., Walravens, K., Roels, S., Meyer, G., Letesson, J.J. and Kerkhofs, P., 2008. Vaccination of calves using the BRSV nucleocapsid protein in a DNA prime-protein boost strategy stimulates cell-mediated immunity and protects the lungs against BRSV replication and pathology, *Vaccine*, 26, 4840-4848.

Letellier, C., Kerkhofs, P., Wellemans, G. and Vanopdenbosch, E., 1999. Detection and genotyping of bovine diarrhea virus by reverse transcription-polymerase chain amplification of the 5' untranslated region, *Veterinary Microbiology*, 64, 155-167.

Li, Y., Van Drunen Littel-Van Den Hurk, Babiuk, L.A. and Liang, X., 1995. Characterization of cell-binding properties of bovine herpesvirus 1 glycoproteins B, C, and D: identification of a dual cell-binding function of gB, *Journal of Virology*, 69, 4758-4768.

Liang, R., van den Hurk, J.V., Landi, A., Lawman, Z., Deregt, D., Townsend, H., Babiuk, L.A. and van Drunen Littel-van den Hurk, 2008. DNA prime protein boost strategies protect cattle from bovine viral diarrhea virus type 2 challenge, *Journal of General Virology*, 89, 453-466.

Liang, X., Pyne, C., Li, Y., Babiuk, L.A. and Kowalski, J., 1995. Delineation of the essential function of bovine herpesvirus 1 gD: an indication for the modulatory role of gD in virus entry, *Virology*, 207, 429-441.

Liebler-Tenorio, E.M., Lanwehr, A., Greiser-Wilke, I., Loehr, B.I. and Pohlenz, J.F., 2000. Comparative investigation of tissue alterations and distribution of BVD-viral antigen in cattle with early onset versus late onset mucosal disease, *Veterinary Microbiology*, 77, 163-174.

Liebler-Tenorio, E.M., Ridpath, J.E. and Neill, J.D., 2002. Distribution of viral antigen and development of lesions after experimental infection with highly virulent bovine viral diarrhea virus type 2 in calves, *American Journal of Veterinary Research*, 63, 1575-1584.

Liess, B. and Moennig, V., 1990. Ruminant pestivirus infection in pigs, *Revue Scientifique et Technique Office International des Epizooties*, 9, 151-161.

Loehr, B.I., Frey, H.R., Moennig, V. and Greiser-Wilke, I., 1998a. Experimental induction of mucosal disease: consequences of superinfection of persistently infected cattle with different strains of cytopathogenic bovine viral diarrhea virus, *Archives of Virology*, 143, 667-679.

Loehr, B.I., Frey, H.R., Moennig, V. and Greiser-Wilke, I., 1998b. [Clinical-virologic course after superinfection of persistently infected cattle with cytopathogenic bovine viral diarrhea virus strains], *Deutsche Tierärztliche Wochenschrift*, 105, 201-204.

Luzzago, C., Piccinini, R., Zepponi, A. and Zecconi, A., 1999. Study on prevalence of bovine viral diarrhoea virus (BVDV) antibodies in 29 Italian dairy herds with reproductive problems, *Veterinary Microbiology*, 64, 247-252.

Madin, S.H., 1956. Isolation of the Infectious Bovine Rhinotracheitis Virus, *Science*, 124, 721-722.

Mahin, L. and Shimi, A., 1982. Weather and BRSV infection, *The Veterinary Record*, 111, 87.

Mahmoud, K., 2007. Recombinant protein production: strategic technology and a vital research tool, *Research Journal Cellular and Molecular Biology*, 1, 9-22.

References

Makoschey, B., 2006. BoHV-1 eradication--one step closer, *Berliner und Münchner Tierärztliche Wochenschrift*, 119, 516-520.

Makoschey, B., Becher, P., Janssen, M.G., Orlich, M., Thiel, H.J. and Lutticken, D., 2004. Bovine viral diarrhea virus with deletions in the 5'-nontranslated region: reduction of replication in calves and induction of protective immunity, *Vaccine*, 22, 3285-3294.

Makoschey, B. and Beer, M., 2004. Assessment of the risk of transmission of vaccine viruses by using insufficiently cleaned injection devices, *The Veterinary Record*, 155, 563-564.

Makoschey, B. and Beer, M., 2007. A live bovine herpesvirus-1 marker vaccine is not shed after intramuscular vaccination, *Berliner und Münchner Tierärztliche Wochenschrift*, 120, 480-482.

Makoschey, B., Chanter, N. and Reddick, D.A., 2006. Comprehensive protection against all important primary pathogens within the bovine respiratory disease complex by combination of two vaccines, *Der Praktische Tierarzt*, 87, 819-826.

Makoschey, B., Donate, J. and Álvarez, M., 2009a. Combined application of an inaCtivated IBR marker vaccine and an inactivated bvd vaccine, *Accepted for publication at the European Buiatrics Forum, December 2009, Marseille, France*.

Makoschey, B., Janssen, M.G., Vrijenhoek, M.P., Korsten, J.H. and Marel, P., 2001. An inactivated bovine virus diarrhoea virus (BVDV) type 1 vaccine affords clinical protection against BVDV type 2, *Vaccine*, 19, 3261-3268.

Makoschey, B. and Janssen, M.G.J., 2009. Investigations on fetal infection models with bovine viral diarrhoea virus (BVDV), *Submitted*.

Makoschey, B. and Keil, G.M., 2000a. Early immunity induced by a glycoprotein E-negative vaccine for infectious bovine rhinotracheitis, *Veterinary Record*, 147, 189-191.

Makoschey, B. and Keil, G.M., 2000b. Early immunity induced by a glycoprotein E-negative vaccine for infectious bovine rhinotracheitis, *The Veterinary Record*, 147, 189-191.

Makoschey, B., Klee, W., Martella, V., Bridger, J., Smiths, D.G., Daugschies, A., Millemann, Y., Liebler-Tenorio, E., Snodgrass, D., Claerebout, E., Bendali, F., van, d., V, Garcia, A., Illek, J., Kaske, M., Cutler, K., Gonzalez-Martin, J.V., Carvalho, L.M., Crouch, C. and Thiry, E., 2009b. Neonatal health in calves--comprehensive solutions for complex enteric disorders, *Berliner und Münchener Tierärztliche Wochenschrift*, 122, 398-408.

Makoschey, B., Liebler-Tenorio, E.M., Biermann, Y.M., Goovaerts, D. and Pohlenz, J.F., 2002a. Leukopenia and thrombocytopenia in pigs after infection with bovine viral diarrhoea virus-2 (BVDV-2), *Deutsche Tierärztliche Wochenschrift*, 109, 225-230.

Makoschey, B., Muñoz Bielsa, J., Catala, M. and Roy, O., 2009c. Experimental safety and efficacy study for the concurrent use of an inactivated bluetongue serotype 8 vaccine with inactivated or live cattle vaccines, *Accepted for publication at the European Buiatrics Forum, December 2009, Marseille, France.*

Makoschey, B., Muñoz Bielsa, J., Oliviëro, L., Roy, O., Pillet, F., Dufe, D., Valla, G. and Cavirani, S., 2008. Efficacy of combination vaccines against bovine respiratory pathogens in calves, *Acta Veterinaria Hungarica*, 56, 485-493.

Makoschey, B., Patel, J.R. and Van Gelder, P.T.J.A., 2002b. Serum-free produced bovine Herpesvirus type 1 and bovine parainfluenza type 3 virus vaccines are efficacious and safe, *Cytotechnology*, 39, 139-145.

Makoschey, B., Sonnemans, D., Bielsa, J.M., Franken, P., Mars, M., Santos, L. and Álvarez, M., 2007a. Evaluation of the induction of NS3 specific BVDV antibodies using a commercial inactivated BVDV vaccine in immunization and challenge trials, *Vaccine*, 25, 6140-6145.

Makoschey, B., van Gelder, P.T., Keijsers, V. and Goovaerts, D., 2003. Bovine viral diarrhoea virus antigen in foetal calf serum batches and consequences of such contamination for vaccine production, *Biologicals*, 31, 203-208.

Makoschey, B., Zehle, H.H., Bussacchini, M., Valla, G., Palfi, V. and Foldi, J., 2007b. Efficacy of a live bovine herpesvirus type 1 marker vaccine under field conditions in three countries, *The Veterinary Record*, 161, 295-298.

Malmquist, W.A., 1968. Bovine viral diarrhea-mucosal disease: Etiology, pathogenesis and applied immunity, *Journal of American Veterinary Medicine Association*, 152, 763-768.

Mandl, C.W., Holzmann, H., Meixner, T., Rauscher, S., Stadler, P.F., Allison, S.L. and Heinz, F.X., 1998. Spontaneous and engineered deletions in the 3' noncoding region of tick-borne encephalitis virus: construction of highly attenuated mutants of a flavivirus, *Journal of Virology*, 72, 2132-2140.

Mannhalter, J.W., Neychev, H.O., Zlabinger, G.J., Ahman, R. and Eibl, M.M., 1985. Modulation of the human immune response by the non-toxic and non-pyrogenic adjuvant aluminium hydroxide: Effect on antigen uptake and antigen presentation, *Clinical and Experimental Immunology*, 61, 143-151.

Marciani, D.J., 2003. Vaccine adjuvants: role and mechanisms of action in vaccine immunogenicity, *Drug Discovery Today*, 8, 934-943.

Mars, M.H., Bruschke, C.J. and Van Oirschot, J.T., 1999. Airborne transmission of BHV1, BRSV, and BVDV among cattle is possible under experimental conditions, *Veterinary Microbiology*, 66, 197-207.

Mars, M.H., de Jong, M.C., Franken, P. and van Oirschot, J.T., 2001. Efficacy of a live glycoprotein E-negative bovine herpesvirus 1 vaccine in cattle in the field, *Vaccine*, 19, 1924-1930.

Mars, M.H., de Jong, M.C. and van Oirschot, J.T., 2000a. A gE-negative BHV1 vaccine virus strain cannot perpetuate in cattle populations, *Vaccine*, 18, 2120-2124.

Mars, M.H., de Jong, M.C. and van Oirschot, J.T., 2000b. A gE-negative bovine herpesvirus 1 vaccine strain is not re-excreted nor transmitted in an experimental cattle population after corticosteroid treatments, *Vaccine*, 18, 1975-1981.

Mars, M.H., Rijsewijk, F.A., Maris-Veldhuis, M.A., Hage, J.J. and van Oirschot, J.T., 2000c. Presence of bovine herpesvirus 1 gB-seropositive but gE-seronegative Dutch cattle with no apparent virus exposure, *The Veterinary Record*, 147, 328-331.

Mars, M.H. and Van Maanen, C., 2005. Diagnostic assays applied in BVDV control in The Netherlands, *Preventive Veterinary Medicine*, 72, 43-48.

Marshall, D.J., Moxley, R.A. and Kelling, C.L., 1996. Distribution of virus and viral antigen in specific pathogen-free calves following inoculation with noncytopathic bovine viral diarrhea virus, *Veterinary Pathology*, 33, 311-318.

Marshall, D.J., Moxley, R.A. and Kelling, C.L., 1998. Severe disease following experimental exposure of calves to noncytopathic bovine viral diarrhoea virus isolate New York-1, *Australian Veterinary Journal*, 76, 428-430.

Maschmann, E., Küster, E. and Fischer, W., 1931. Über die Fähigkeit des Tonerde-Präparates B, Diphtherie-Toxin zu adsorbieren., *Berichte derDeutschen Chemiker Gesellschaft*, 64, 2174-2178.

Mawhinney, I. and Makoschey, B., 2008. Compatibility of inactivated bovine viral diarrhoea (BVD) and *Leptospira interrogans serovar hardjo* vaccines, *World Buiatric Congress, Budapest, 2008*.

Mawhinney, I., Watson, C. and Patel, J.R., 2007. Seroprevalence of BVDV in cattle of different age groups on 17 dairy farms in the West of England, *The Veterinary Record*, 160, 738-740.

Mawhinney, I.C. and Burrows, M.R., 2005. Protection against bovine respiratory syncytial virus challenge following a single dose of vaccine in young calves with maternal antibody, *The Veterinary Record*, 156, 139-143.

McGowan, M.R., Kafi, M., Kirkland, P.D., Kelly, R., Bielefeldt-Ohmann, H., Occhio, M.D. and Jillella, D., 2003. Studies of the pathogenesis of bovine pestivirus-induced ovarian dysfunction in superovulated dairy cattle, *Theriogenology*, 59, 1051-1066.

McGowan, M.R., Kirkland, P.D., Richards, S.G. and Littlejohns, I.R., 1993. Increased reproductive losses in cattle infected with bovine pestivirus around the time of insemination, *The Veterinary Record*, 133, 39-43.

Meehan, J.T., Lehmkuhl, H.D., Cutlip, R.C. and Bolin, S.R., 1998. Acute pulmonary lesions in sheep experimentally infected with bovine viral diarrhoea virus, *Journal of Comparative Pathology*, 119, 277-292.

Men, R., Bray, M., Clark, D., Chanock, R.M. and Lai, C.J., 1996. Dengue type 4 virus mutants containing deletions in the 3' noncoding region of the RNA genome: analysis of growth restriction in cell culture and altered viremia pattern and immunogenicity in rhesus monkeys, *Journal of Virology*, 70, 3930-3937.

Mett, V., Farrance, C.E., Green, B.J. and Yusibov, V., 2008. Plants as biofactories, *Biologicals*, 36, 354-358.

Metzler, A.E., Schudel, A.A. and Engels, M., 1986. Bovine herpesvirus 1: Molecular and antigenic characteristics of variant viruses isolated from calves with neurological disease, *Archives of Virology*, 87, 205-217.

Meyers, G. and Thiel, H.J., 1996. Molecular characterization of pestiviruses, *Advances In Virus Research*, 47, 53-118.

Meyling, A. and Jensen, A.M., 1988. Transmission of bovine virus diarrhoea virus (BVDV) by artificial insemination (AI) with semen from a persistently-infected bull, *Veterinary Microbiology*, 17, 97-105.

Moen, A., Sol, J. and Sampimon, O., 2005. Indication of transmission of BVDV in the absence of persistently infected (PI) animals, *Preventive Veterinary Medicine*, 72, 93-98.

Moennig, V., Eicken, K., Flebbe, U., Frey, H.R., Grummer, B., Haas, L., Greiser-Wilke, I. and Liess, B., 2005a. Implementation of two-step vaccination in the control of bovine viral diarrhoea (BVD), *Preventive Veterinary Medicine*, 72, 109-114.

Moennig, V., Houe, H. and Lindberg, A., 2005b. BVD control in Europe: current status and perspectives, *Animal Health Research Review*, 6, 63-74.

Moennig, V. and Liess, B., 1995. Pathogenesis of intrauterine infections with bovine viral diarrhea virus, *Veterinary clinics of North Amerika: food animal practice*, 11, 477-487.

Moennig, V. and Plagemann, P.G., 1992. The pestiviruses, *Advances In Virus Research*, 41, 53-98.

Moerman, A., Straver, P.J., De Jong, M.C., Quak, J., Baanvinger, T. and van Oirschot, J.T., 1994. Clinical consequences of a bovine virus diarrhoea virus infection in a dairy herd: a longitudinal study, *Veterinary Quarterly*, 16, 115-119.

Monaco, F., Camma, C., Serini, S. and Savini, G., 2006. Differentiation between field and vaccine strain of bluetongue virus serotype 16, *Veterinary Microbiology*, 116, 45-52.

Moran, E., 1999. A microcarrier-based cell culture process for the production of a bovine respiratory syncytial virus vaccine, *Cytotechnology*, 29, 135-148.

Morzaria, S.P., Richards, M.S., Harkness, J.W. and Maund, B.A., 1979. A field trial with a multicomponent inactivated respiratory viral vaccine, *The Veterinary Record*, 105, 410-414.

Muylkens, B., Meurens, F., Schynts, F., Farnir, F., Pourchet, A., Bardiau, M., Gogev, S., Thiry, J., Cuisenaire, A., Vanderplasschen, A. and Thiry, E., 2006. Intraspecific bovine herpesvirus 1 recombinants carrying glycoprotein E deletion as a vaccine marker are virulent in cattle, *Journal of General Virology*, 87, 2149-2154.

Nicholson, K.G., 2009. Influenza and vaccine development: a continued battle, *Expert Review of Vaccines*, 8, 373-374.

Niskanen, R. and Lindberg, A., 2003. Transmission of bovine viral diarrhoea virus by unhygienic vaccination procedures, ambient air, and from contaminated pens, *The Veterinary Journal*, 165, 125-130.

Niskanen, R., Lindberg, A., Larsson, B. and Alenius, S., 2000. Lack of virus transmission from bovine viral diarrhoea virus infected calves to susceptible peers, *Acta Veterinaria Scandinavia*, 41, 93-99.

Niskanen, R., Lindberg, A. and Traven, M., 2002. Failure to spread bovine virus diarrhoea virus infection from primarily infected calves despite concurrent infection with bovine coronavirus, *The Veterinary Journal*, 163, 251-259.

O'Toole, D., Van Campen, H. and Woodard, L., 1994. Bluetongue virus: contamination of vaccine, *Journal of the American Veterinary Medical Association*, 205, 407-408.

Odeon, A.C., Kelling, C.L., Marshall, D.J., Estela, E.S., Dubovi, E.J. and Donis, R.O., 1999. Experimental infection of calves with bovine viral diarrhea virus genotype II (NY-93), *Journal of Veterinary Diagnostic Investigation*, 11, 221-228.

Olafson, P., MacCallum, A.D. and Fox, F.H., 1946. An apparently new transmissible disease of cattle, *The Cornell veterinarian*, 36, 205-213.

Olmsted, R.A., Elango, N., Prince, G.A., Murphy, B.R., Johnson, P.R., Moss, B., Chanock, R.M. and Collins, P.L., 1986. Expression of the F glycoprotein of respiratory syncytial virus by a recombinant vaccinia virus: comparison of the individual contributions of the F and G glycoproteins to host immunity, *Proceedings of the National Academy of Sciences USA*, 83, 7462-7466.

Openshaw, P.J. and Tregoning, J.S., 2005. Immune responses and disease enhancement during respiratory syncytial virus infection, *Clinical Microbiology Reviews*, 18, 541-555.

Parsonson, I.M., 1990. Pathology and pathogenesis of bluetongue infections, *Current Topics in Microbiology and Immunology*, 162, 119-141.

Passler, T., Walz, P.H., Ditchkoff, S.S., Brock, K.V., Deyoung, R.W., Foley, A.M. and Daniel, G.M., 2009. Cohabitation of pregnant white-tailed deer and cattle persistently infected with Bovine viral diarrhea virus results in persistently infected fawns, *Veterinary Microbiology*, 134, 362-367.

Pastey, M.K. and Samal, S.K., 1995. Nucleotide sequence analysis of the non-structural NS1 (1C) and NS2 (1B) protein genes of bovine respiratory syncytial virus, *Journal of General Virology*, 76 (Pt 1), 193-197.

References

Pastey, M.K. and Samal, S.K., 1997. Role of individual N-linked oligosaccharide chains and different regions of bovine respiratory syncytial virus fusion protein in cell surface transport, *Archives of Virology*, 142, 2309-2320.

Pastoret, P.P., Thiry, E., Brochier, B. and Derboven, G., 1982. Bovid herpesvirus 1 infection of cattle: pathogenesis, latency, consequences of latency, *Annales de recherches vétérinaires*, 13, 221-235.

Patel, J.R., 2004. Evaluation of a quadrivalent inactivated vaccine for the protection of cattle against diseases due to common viral infections, *Journal of the South African Veterinary Association*, 75, 137-146.

Patel, J.R., Didlick, S. and Brunner, R., 2004. Untersuchungen mit einem IBR-Marker-Lebendimpfstoff zum Nachweis eines vereinfachten Impfschemas (Grundimmunisierung durch Einmalimpfung), *Tierärztliche Umschau*, 59, 583-586.

Patel, J.R., Didlick, S. and Quinton, J., 2005. Variation in immunogenicity of ruminant pestiviruses as determined by the neutralisation assay, *The Veterinary Journal*, 169, 468-472.

Patel, J.R. and Shilleto, R.W., 2005. Modification of active immunization with live bovine herpesvirus 1 vaccine by passive viral antibody, *Vaccine*, 23, 4023-4028.

Patel, J.R., Shilleto, R.W., Williams, J. and Alexander, D.C., 2002. Prevention of transplacental infection of bovine foetus by bovine viral diarrhoea virus through vaccination, *Archives of Virology*, 147, 2453-2463.

Patil, P.K., Bayry, J., Ramakrishna, C., Hugar, B., Misra, L.D., Prabhudas, K. and Natarajan, C., 2002. Immune responses of sheep to quadrivalent double emulsion foot-and-mouth disease vaccines: rate of development of immunity and variations among other ruminants, *Journal of Clinical Microbiology*, 40, 4367-4371.

Paton, D.J., 1995. Pestivirus diversity, *Journal of Comparative Pathology*, 112, 215-236.

Paton, D.J., Ibata, G., Edwards, S. and Wensvoort, G., 1991. An ELISA detecting antibody to conserved pestivirus epitopes, *Journal of Virological Methods*, 31, 315-324.

Peterhans, E., Jungi, T.W. and Schweizer, M., 2003. BVDV and innate immunity, *Biologicals*, 31, 107-112.

Peters, A.R., Thevasagayam, S.J., Wiseman, A. and Salt, J.S., 2004. Duration of immunity of a quadrivalent vaccine against respiratory diseases caused by BHV-1, PI(3)V, BVDV, and BRSV in experimentally infected calves, *Preventive Veterinary Medicine*, 66, 63-77.

Petrini, S., Ramadori, G., Corradi, A., Borghetti, P., Lombardi, G., Villa, R., Bottarelli, E., Guercio, A., Amici, A. and Ferrari, M., Evaluation of safety and efficacy of DNA vaccines against bovine herpesvirus-1 (BoHV-1) in calves, *Comparative Immunology, Microbiology and Infectious Diseases*, In Press, Corrected Proof.

References

Platt, R., Burdett, W. and Roth, J.A., 2006. Induction of antigen-specific T-cell subset activation to bovine respiratory disease viruses by a modified-live virus vaccine, *Amerian Journal of Veterinary Research*, 67, 1179-1184.

Platt, R., Coutu, C., Meinert, T. and Roth, J.A., 2008. Humoral and T cell-mediated immune responses to bivalent killed bovine viral diarrhea virus vaccine in beef cattle, *Veterinary Immunology and Immunopathology*, 122, 8-15.

Platt, R., Widel, P.W., Kesl, L.D. and Roth, J.A., 2009. Comparison of humoral and cellular immune responses to a pentavalent modified live virus vaccine in three age groups of calves with maternal antibodies, before and after BVDV type 2 challenge, *Vaccine*, 27, 4508-4519.

Plotkin, S.A., Cadoz, M., Meignier, B., Meric, C., Leroy, O., Excler, J.L., Tartaglia, J., Paoletti, E., Gonczol, E. and Chappuis, G., 1995. The safety and use of canarypox vectored vaccines, *Developments in biological standardization*, 84, 165-170.

Plowright, W. and Ferris, R.D., 1962. Studies with rinderpest virus in tissue culture. The use of attenuate culture virus as a vaccine for cattle, *Research in Veterinary Science*, 3, 172-182.

Polak, M.P. and Zmudzinski, J.F., 2000. Experimental inoculation of calves with laboratory strains of bovine viral diarrhea virus, *Comparitive Immunology Microbiology and Infectious Diseases.*, 23, 141-151.

Potgieter, L.N.D., 1995. Immunology of bovine viral diarrhea virus, *Veterinary clinics of North Amerika: food animal practice*, 11, 501-520.

Potgieter, L.N.D., McCracken, M.d., Hopkins, F.M. and Guy J.S., 1985. Comparison of pneumopathogenicity of two strains of bovine viral diarrhea virus, *American Journal of Veterinary Research*, 46, 151-153.

Presi, P. and Heim, D., BVD eradication in Switzerland--A new approach, *Veterinary Microbiology*, In Press, Corrected Proof.

Rabenau, H., Ohlinger, V., Anderson, J., Selb, B., Cinatl, J., Wolf, W., Frost, J., Mellor, P. and Doerr, H.W., 1993. Contamination of genetically engineered CHO-cells by epizootic haemorrhagic disease virus (EHDV), *Biologicals*, 21, 207-214.

Rai, M. and Padh, H., 2001. Expression systems for production of heterologous proteins, *Current Science*, 80, 1121-1128.

Raleigh, P., 2007. Foot & Mouth outbreak linked to process failings, *Process Engineering (London)*, 88, 9.

Ramsey, F.K. and Chivers, W.H., 1953. Mucosal disease of cattle, *The North American veterinarian*, 34, 629-633.

Reber, A.J., Tanner, M., Okinaga, T., Woolums, A.R., Williams, S., Ensley, D.T. and Hurley, D.J., 2006. Evaluation of multiple immune parameters after vaccination with modified live or killed bovine viral diarrhea virus vaccines, *Comparative Immunology Microbiology and Infectious Diseases.*, 29, 61-77.

Rebhun, W.C., French, T.W., Perdrizet, J.A., Dubovi, E., Dill, S.G. and Karcher, L.F., 1989. Thrombocytopenia associated with acute bovine virus diarrhea infection in cattle, *Journal of Veterinary Internal Medicine*, 3, 42-46.

Reimann, I., Semmler, I. and Beer, M., 2007. Packaged replicons of bovine viral diarrhea virus are capable of inducing a protective immune response, *Virology*, 366, 377-386.

Reisinger, L. and Reimann, H., 1928. Beitrag zur Äthiologie des Bläschenausschlages des Rindes, *Wiener Tierärztliche Monatsschrift*, 15, 249-261.

Ridpath, J.E., Neill, J.D., Endsley, J. and Roth, J.A., 2003. Effect of passive immunity on the development of a protective immune response against bovine viral diarrhea virus in calves, *American Journal of Veterinary Research*, 64, 65-69.

Ridpath, J.F., Bolin, S.R. and Dubovi, E.J., 1994. Segregation of bovine viral diarrhea virus into genotypes, *Virology*, 205, 66-74.

Ridpath, J.F., Neill, J.D. and Peterhans, E., 2007. Impact of variation in acute virulence of BVDV1 strains on design of better vaccine efficacy challenge models, *Vaccine*, 25, 8058-8066.

Rijsewijk, F.A.M., Kaashoek, M.J., Langeveld, J.P.M., Meloen, R., Judek, J., Bienkowska-Szewczyk, K., Maris-Veldhuis, M.A. and van Oirschot, J.T., 1999. Epitopes on glycoprotein C of bovine herpesvirus-1 (BHV-1) that allow differentiation between BHV-1.1 and BHV-1.2 strains, *Journal of General Virology*, 80, 1477-1483.

Rikula, U., Nuotio, L., Laamanen, U.I. and Sihvonen, L., 2008. Transmission of bovine viral diarrhoea virus through the semen of acutely infected bulls under field conditions, *The Veterinary Record*, 162, 79-81.

Rissi, D.R., Pierezan, F., Silva, M.S., Flores, E.F. and de Barros, C.S., 2008. Neurological disease in cattle in southern Brazil associated with Bovine herpesvirus infection, *Journal of Veterinary Diagnostic Investigation*, 20, 346-349.

Robinson, K.E., Meers, J., Gravel, J.L., McCarthy, F.M. and Mahony, T.J., 2008. The essential and non-essential genes of Bovine herpesvirus 1, *Journal of General Virology*, 89, 2851-2863.

Rosas, C.T., Konig, P., Beer, M., Dubovi, E.J., Tischer, B.K. and Osterrieder, N., 2007. Evaluation of the vaccine potential of an equine herpesvirus type 1 vector expressing bovine viral diarrhea virus structural proteins, *Journal of General Virology*, 88, 748-757.

Rüfenacht, J., Schaller, P., Audige, L., Knutti, B., Kupfer, U. and Peterhans, E., 2001. The effect of infection with bovine viral diarrhea virus on the fertility of Swiss dairy cattle, *Theriogenology*, 56, 199-210.

Sandvik, T., 2004. Progress of control and prevention programs for bovine viral diarrhea virus in Europe, *Veterinary clinics of North Amerika: food animal practice*, 20, 151-169.

References

Schelp, C., Greiser-Wilke, I. and Moennig, V., 2000. An actin-binding protein is involved in pestivirus entry into bovine cells, *Virus Research*, 68, 1-5.

Schlender, J., Bossert, B., Buchholz, U. and Conzelmann, K.K., 2000. Bovine respiratory syncytial virus nonstructural proteins NS1 and NS2 cooperatively antagonize alpha/beta interferon-induced antiviral response, *Journal of Virology*, 74, 8234-8242.

Schlender, J., Walliser, G., Fricke, J. and Conzelmann, K.K., 2002. Respiratory syncytial virus fusion protein mediates inhibition of mitogen-induced T-cell proliferation by contact, *Journal of Virology*, 76, 1163-1170.

Schlender, J., Zimmer, G., Herrler, G. and Conzelmann, K.K., 2003. Respiratory syncytial virus (RSV) fusion protein subunit F2, not attachment protein G, determines the specificity of RSV infection, *Journal of Virology*, 77, 4609-4616.

Schmidt, U., Beyer, J., Polster, U., Gershwin, L.J. and Buchholz, U.J., 2002. Mucosal immunization with live recombinant bovine respiratory syncytial virus (BRSV) and recombinant BRSV lacking the envelope glycoprotein G protects against challenge with wild-type BRSV, *Journal of Virology*, 76, 12355-12359.

Schneider, R., Unger, G., Stark, R., Schneider-Scherzer, E. and Thiel, H.J., 1993. Identification of a structural glycoprotein of an RNA virus as a ribonuclease, *Science*, 261, 1169-1171.

Schreiber, P., Matheise, J.P., Dessy, F., Heimann, M., Letesson, J.J., Coppe, P. and Collard, A., 2000. High mortality rate associated with bovine respiratory syncytial virus (BRSV) infection in Belgian white blue calves previously vaccinated with an inactivated BRSV vaccine, *Journal of Veterinary Medicine, Series B*, 47, 535-550.

Schroeder, R.J. and Moys, M.D., 1954. An upper respiratory infection in dairy cattle, *Journal of the American Veterinary Medical Association*, 125, 471.

Senda, M., Parrish, C.R., Harasawa, R., Gamoh, K., Muramatsu, M., Hirayama, N. and Itoh, O., 1995. Detection by PCR of wild-type canine parvovirus which contaminates dog vaccines, *Journal of Clinical Microbiology*, 33, 110-113.

Spinage, C.A. 2004. The final European Outbreaks. In: *Cattle Plague: a History*, pp. 189-216.

Stalder, H.P., Meier, P., Pfaffen, G., Wageck-Canal, C., Rufenacht, J., Schaller, P., Bachofen, C., Marti, S., Vogt, H.R. and Peterhans, E., 2005. Genetic heterogeneity of pestiviruses of ruminants in Switzerland, *Preventive Veterinary Medicine*, 72, 37-41.

Stott, E.J., Ball, L.A., Young, K.K., Furze, J. and Wertz, G.W., 1986. Human respiratory syncytial virus glycoprotein G expressed from a recombinant vaccinia virus vector protects mice against live-virus challenge, *Journal of Virology*, 60, 607-613.

Stott, E.J., Thomas, L.H., Collins, A.P., Crouch, S., Jebbet, N.J., Smith, G.S., Luther, P.D. and Caswell, R., 1980. A survey of virus infections of the respiratory tract of cattle and their association with disease, *Journal of Hygiene*, 85, 257-270.

Stott, E.J., Thomas, L.H., Howard, C.J. and Gourlay, R.N., 1987. Field trial of a quadrivalent vaccine against calf respiratory disease, *The Veterinary Record*, 121, 342-347.

Straub, O.C., 1978. Vorkommen der durch IBR-IPV-Viren hervorgerufenen Krankheiten und mögliche Differentialdiagnostische Probleme in den verschiedenen Kontinenten und deren Länder, *Deutsche Tierärztliche Wochenschrift*, 85, 84-90.

Straub, O.C. 1990. Infectious Bovine Rhinotracheitis Virus. In: *Virus Infections of Ruminants* (Ed. by Z.Dinter & B.Morein), pp. 71-150. Amsterdam, Elsevier Science Publishers B.V.

Tajima, M., Frey, H., Yamato, O., Maede, Y., Moennig, V., Scholz, H. and Greiser-Wilke, I., 2001. Prevalence of genotypes 1 and 2 of bovine viral diarrhea virus in Lower Saxony, Germany, *Virus Research*, 76, 31-42.

Tajima, M., Yuasa, M., Kawanabe, M., Taniyama, H., Yamato, O. and Maede, Y., 1999. Possible causes of diabetes mellitus in cattle infected with bovine viral diarroea virus, *Journal of Veterinary Medicine B*, 46, 207-215.

Tautz, N., Meyers, G. and Thiel, H.J., 1998. Pathogenesis of mucosal disease, a deadly disease of cattle caused by a pestivirus, *Clinical and Diagnostic Virology*, 10, 121-127.

Taylor, G., Bruce, C., Barbet, A.F., Wyld, S.G. and Thomas, L.H., 2005. DNA vaccination against respiratory syncytial virus in young calves, *Vaccine*, 23, 1242-1250.

Taylor, G., Rijsewijk, F.A., Thomas, L.H., Wyld, S.G., Gaddum, R.M., Cook, R.S., Morrison, W.I., Hensen, E., Van Oirschot, J.T. and Keil, G., 1998. Resistance to bovine respiratory syncytial virus (BRSV) induced in calves by a recombinant bovine herpesvirus-1 expressing the attachment glycoprotein of BRSV, *Journal of General Virology*, 79, 1759-1767.

Taylor, G., Thomas, L.H., Furze, J.M., Cook, R.S., Wyld, S.G., Lerch, R., Hardy, R. and Wertz, G.W., 1997. Recombinant vaccinia viruses expressing the F, G or N, but not the M2 protein of bovine respiratory syncytial virus (BRVS) induce resistance to BRSV challenge in the calf and protect against the development of pneumonic lesions, *Journal of General Virology*, 78, 3195-3206.

Taylor, G., Thomas, L.H., Wyld, S.G., Furze, J., Sopp, P. and Howard, C.J., 1995. Role of T-lymphocyte subsets in recovery from respiratory syncytial virus infection in calves, *Journal of Virology*, 69, 6658-6664.

The European agency for the evaluation of medicinal products veterinary medicines and inspections, 2002. Guideline on requirements and controls applied to bovine serum used in the production of immunological veterinary products, EMEA/CVMP/743/00.

The European Directorate for the Quality of Medicines & Health Care 2009. Bovine viral diarrhoea vaccine (inactivated) [Vaccinum diarrhoeae viralis bovinae inactivatum]. In: *European Pharmacopoeia 6.0*.

References

Thiel, H.-J., 1996. Molecular Characterization of Pestiviruses, *Advances In Virus Research* 47, 53-118.

Thiry, E., Muylkens, B., Meurens, F., Gogev, S., Thiry, J., Vanderplasschen, A. and Schynts, F., 2006a. Recombination in the alphaherpesvirus bovine herpesvirus 1, *Veterinary Microbiology*, 113, 171-177.

Thiry, J., Keuser, V., Muylkens, B., Meurens, F., Gogev, S., Vanderplasschen, A. and Thiry, E., 2006b. Ruminant alphaherpesviruses related to bovine herpesvirus 1, *Veterinary Research*, 37, 169-190.

Thiry, J., Tempesta, M., Camero, M., Tarsitano, E., Muylkens, B., Meurens, F., Thiry, E. and Buonavoglia, C., 2007. Clinical protection against caprine herpesvirus 1 genital infection by intranasal administration of a live attenuated glycoprotein E negative bovine herpesvirus 1 vaccine, *BMC Veterinary Research*, 3, 33.

Thomas, C., Young, N.J., Heaney, J., Collins, M.E. and Brownlie, J., 2009. Evaluation of efficacy of mammalian and baculovirus expressed E2 subunit vaccine candidates to bovine viral diarrhoea virus, *Vaccine*, 27, 2387-2393.

Thomas, L.H., Stott, E.J., Collins, A.P., Jebbet, N.J. and Stark, A.J., 1977. Evaluation of respiratory disease in calves: Comparison of disease response to different viruses, *Research in Veterinary Science*, 23, 157-164.

Thomas, L.H., Stott, E.J., Collins, A.P. and Jebbett, J., 1984. Experimental pneumonia in gnotobiotic calves produced by respiratory syncytial virus, *British journal of experimental pathology*, 65, 19-28.

Tikoo, S.K., Campos, M. and Babiuk, L.A., 1995. Bovine herpesvirus 1 (BHV-1): biology, pathogenesis, and control, *Advances in Virus Research*, 45, 191-223.

Topliff, C.L. and Kelling, C.L., 1998. Virulence Markers in the 5' Untranslated Region of Genotype 2 Bovine Viral diarrhea Virus isolates, *Virology*, 250, 164-172.

Toth, R.L., Nettleton, P.F. and McCrae, M.A., 1999. Expression of the E2 envelope glycoprotein of bovine viral diarrhoea virus (BVDV) elicits virus-type specific neutralising antibodies, *Veterinary Microbiology*, 65, 87-101.

Trapp, S., Osterrieder, N., Keil, G.M. and Beer, M., 2003. Mutagenesis of a bovine herpesvirus type 1 genome cloned as an infectious bacterial artificial chromosome: analysis of glycoprotein E and G double deletion mutants, *Journal of General Virology*, 84, 301-306.

United States Department of Agriculture, 2002. Center for Veterinary Biologics Notice No. 02-19 (Vaccine Claims for Protection of the Fetus Against Bovine Virus Diarrhea Virus), http://www.aphis.usda.gov/animal_health/vet_biologics/publications.

Valarcher, J.F., Bourhy, H., Lavenu, A., Bourges-Abella, N., Roth, M., Andreoletti, O., Ave, P. and Schelcher, F., 2001. Persistent Infection of B Lymphocytes by Bovine Respiratory Syncytial Virus, *Virology*, 291, 55-67.

Valarcher, J.F., Furze, J., Wyld, S.G., Cook, R., Zimmer, G., Herrler, G. and Taylor, G., 2006. Bovine respiratory syncytial virus lacking the virokinin or with a mutation in furin cleavage site RA(R/K)R109 induces less pulmonary inflammation without impeding the induction of protective immunity in calves, *Journal of General Virology*, 87, 1659-1667.

Valarcher, J.F., Schelcher, F. and Bourhy, H., 2000. Evolution of bovine respiratory syncytial virus [In Process Citation], *Journal of Virology*, 74, 10714-10728.

Valarcher, J.F. and Taylor, G., 2007. Bovine respiratory syncytial virus infection, *Veterinary Research*, 38, 153-180.

Van Campen, H., 2009. Epidemiology and control of BVD in the U.S, *Veterinary Microbiology*, In Press, Corrected Proof.

Van der Poel, W.H.M., Kramps, J.A., Middel, W.G., Van Oirschot, J.T. and Brand, A., 1993. Dynamics of bovine respiratory syncytial virus infections: a longitudinal epidemiological study in dairy herds, *Archives of Virology*, 133, 309-321.

Van der Poel, W.H.M., Langedijk, J.P., Kramps, J.A., Middel, W.G., Brand, A. and Van Oirschot, J.T., 1997. Serological indication for persistence of bovine respiratory syncytial virus in cattle and attempts to detect the virus, *Archives of Virology*, 142, 1681-1696.

van der Sluijs, M.T.W., Kuhn, E.M. and Makoschey, B., 2009. A single vaccination with an inactivated bovine respiratory syncytial virus vaccine primes the cellular immune response in calves with maternal antibodies, *BMC Veterinary Research*, Accepted.

Van Drunen Littel-Van Den Hurk, Loehr, B.I. and Babiuk, L.A., 2001. Immunization of livestock with DNA vaccines: current studies and future prospects, *Vaccine*, 19, 2474-2479.

Van Drunen Littel-Van Den Hurk, Snider, M., Thompson, P., Latimer, L. and Babiuk, L.A., 2008. Strategies for induction of protective immunity to bovine herpesvirus-1 in newborn calves with maternal antibodies, *Vaccine*, 26, 3103-3111.

van Drunen, L., Braun, R.P., Lewis, P.J., Karvonen, B.C., Baca-Estrada, M.E., Snider, M., McCartney, D., Watts, T. and Babiuk, L.A., 1998. Intradermal immunization with a bovine herpesvirus-1 DNA vaccine induces protective immunity in cattle, *Journal of General Virology*, 79, 831-839.

van Engelenburg, F.A., Kaashoek, M.J., van Oirschot, J.T. and Rijsewijk, F.A., 1995. A glycoprotein E deletion mutant of bovine herpesvirus 1 infects the same limited number of tissues in calves as wild-type virus, but for a shorter period, *Journal of General Virology*, 76 (Pt 9), 2387-2392.

van Oirschot, J.T., 1999. Bovine viral vaccines, diagnostics, and eradication: past, present, and future, *Advances in Veterianry Medicine*, 41, 197-216.

Van Oirschot, J.T., 1999. Diva vaccines that reduce virus transmission, *J. Biotechnol.*, 73, 195-205.

van Oirschot, J.T., Gielkens, A.L., Moormann, R.J. and Berns, A.J., 1990. Marker vaccines, virus protein-specific antibody assays and the control of Aujeszky's disease, *Veterinary Microbiology*, 23, 85-101.

Vangeel, I., Antonis, A.F.G., Fluess, M., Peters, A.R. and Harmeyer, S.S., 2005. Efficacy of a modified live bovine respiratory syncytial virus vaccine in three-week-old calve experimentally challenged with BRSV, *Cattle Practice*, 13, 263-271.

Veits, J., Wiesner, D., Fuchs, W., Hoffmann, B., Granzow, H., Starick, E., Mundt, E., Schirrmeier, H., Mebatsion, T., Mettenleiter, T.C. and Romer-Oberdorfer, A., 2006. Newcastle disease virus expressing H5 hemagglutinin gene protects chickens against Newcastle disease and avian influenza, *Proceedings of the National Academy of Science U. S. A*, 103, 8197-8202.

Vilcek, S., Durkovic, B., Kolesarova, M. and Paton, D.J., 2005. Genetic diversity of BVDV: consequences for classification and molecular epidemiology, *Preventive Veterinary Medicine*, 72, 31-35.

Viuff, B., Larsen, L.E., Rontved, C.M., Uttenthal, A., Ronsholt, L. and Alexandersen, S., 2002. Replication and clearance of respiratory syncytial virus: apoptosis is an important pathway of virus clearance after experimental infection with bovine respiratory syncytial virus, *Amercan journal of pathology*, 161, 2195-2207.

Viuff, B., Uttenthal, A., Tegtmeier, C. and Alexandersen, S., 1996. Sites of replication of bovine respiratory syncytial virus in naturally infected calves as determined by in situ hybridization, *Veterinary Pathology*, 33, 383-390.

Waldmann, D., Kobe, K. and Pyl, G., 1937. Die aktive Immunisierung des Rindes gegen Maul- und Klauenseuche., *Zentralblatt Bakteriologie Origin.*, 138, 401.

Walz, P.H., Bell, T.G., Wells, J.L., Grooms, D.L., Kaiser, L., Maes, R.K. and Baker, J.C., 2001. Relationship between degree of viremia and disease manifestation in calves with experimentally induced bovine viral diarrhea virus infection, *American Journal of Veterinary Research*, 62, 1095-1103.

Weiland, E., Stark, R., Haas, B., Rumenapf, T., Meyers, G. and Thiel, H.J., 1990. Pestivirus glycoprotein which induces neutralizing antibodies forms part of a disulfide-linked heterodimer, *Journal of Virology*, 64, 3563-3569.

West, K., Petrie, L., Haines, D.M., Konoby, C., Clark, E.G., Martin, K. and Ellis, J.A., 1999a. The effect of formalin-inactivated vaccine on respiratory disease associated with bovine respiratory syncytial virus infection in calves, *Vaccine*, 17, 809-820.

West, K., Petrie, L., Konoby, C., Haines, D.M., Cortese, V. and Ellis, J.A., 1999b. The efficacy of modified-live bovine respiratory syncytial virus vaccines in experimentally infected calves, *Vaccine*, 18, 907-919.

Whitehead, S.S., Bukreyev, A., Teng, M.N., Firestone, C.Y., St Claire, M., Elkins, W.R., Collins, P.L. and Murphy, B.R., 1999. Recombinant respiratory syncytial virus bearing a deletion of either the NS2 or SH gene is attenuated in chimpanzees, *Journal of Virology*, 73, 3438-3442.

Wiktor, T.J., Aalestad, H.G. and Kaplan, M.M., 1972. Immunogenicity of rabies virus inactivated by ß-propopiolactone, acetylethylenimine, and ionizing irradiation, *Applied Microbiology*, 23, 914-918.

Winkler, M.T., Doster, A. and Jones, C., 1999. Bovine herpesvirus 1 can infect CD4(+) T lymphocytes and induce programmed cell death during acute infection of cattle, *Journal of Virology*, 73, 8657-8668.

Wolfmeyer, A., Wolf, G., Beer, M., Strube, W., Hehnen, H.R., Schmeer, N. and Kaaden, O.-R., 1997. Genomic (5'UTR) and serological differences among Germany BVDV field isolates, *Archives of Virology*, 142, 2049-2057.

World Organization for Animal Health, 2009. Handistatus II, http://www.oie.int/hs2/report.asp .

Xue, W. and Minocha, H.C., 1993. Identification of the cell surface receptor for bovine viral diarrhoea virus by using anti-idiotypic antibodies, *Journal of General Virology*, 74, 73-79.

Zhang, L., Peeples, M.E., Boucher, R.C., Collins, P.L. and Pickles, R.J., 2002. Respiratory syncytial virus infection of human airway epithelial cells is polarized, specific to ciliated cells, and without obvious cytopathology, *Journal of Virology*, 76, 5654-5666.

Zhang, W., Inan, M. and Meagher, M.M., 2000. Fermentation strategies for recombinant protein expression in the methylotrophic yeast Pichia pastoris, *Biotechnology and Bioprocess Engineering*, 5, 275-287.

Zimmer, G., Rohn, M., McGregor, G.P., Schemann, M., Conzelmann, K.K. and Herrler, G., 2003. Virokinin, a bioactive peptide of the tachykinin family, is released from the fusion protein of bovine respiratory syncytial virus, *The Journal of biological chemistry*, 278, 46854-46861.

Zimmer, G.M., Wentink, G.H., Bruschke, C., Westenbrink, F.J., Brinkhof, J. and de, G., I, 2002. Failure of foetal protection after vaccination against an experimental infection with bovine virus diarrhea virus, *Veterinary Microbiology*, 89, 255-265.

Anhang

Publikationen, die Bestandteil der Habilitationsschrift sind:

An inactivated bovine virus diarrhoea virus (BVDV) type 1 vaccine affords clinical protection against BVDV type 2
Makoschey, B.; Janssen, M.G.J.; Vrijenhoek, M.P.; Korsten, J.H.M. and van der Marel, P. (2001)
Vaccine 19, 3261-3268

This study was designed to answer to two distinct questions. Firstly, is it possible to reproduce clinical signs of acute bovine virus diarrhoea virus (BVDV) type 2 infection including signs of haemorrhagic disease under experimental conditions in cattle at 20 weeks of age? Secondly, what is the extent of the protection afforded by vaccination with an inactivated BVDV type 1 vaccine against BVDV type 2 infection? Calves were vaccinated at 12 and 16 weeks of age with a commercially available inactivated BVDV type 1 vaccine (Bovilis BVD). At 20 weeks they were challenge infected with BVDV type 2 virus together with unvaccinated control calves. The unvaccinated animals developed typical signs of respiratory disease, diarrhoea with erosions and haemorrhages along the whole length gastro-intestinal tract, and depletion of lymphocytes in lymphatic organs. These signs were either absent or markedly less severe in the vaccinated animals. The beneficial effects of vaccination were most striking in the haematological parameters thrombocytopenia and leukopenia. It can be concluded that vaccination with Bovilis BVD affords cross-protection against clinical effects of a challenge-infection with heterologous type 2 BVDV.

Bovine viral diarrhoea virus antigen in foetal calf serum batches and consequences of such contamination for vaccine production
Makoschey, B., van Gelder, P.T., Keijsers, V. and Goovaerts, D. (2003)
Biologicals, 31, 203-208

A protocol to test foetal calf serum (FCS) for contamination with bovine viral diarrhoea virus (BVDV) is described. Following this protocol, which combines cell culture methods and detection of pestivirus RNA, seven batches of FCS were tested. Infectious BVDV was detected in four of those batches. One of the remaining batches contained a relatively high number of non-infectious BVDV particles. A sample of this batch was formulated with aluminium hydroxide and aluminium phosphate as adjuvant into an experimental vaccine preparation. This product was injected twice into BVDV seronegative cattle with a 4 week interval. Blood samples taken 4 weeks after the second application were negative for BVDV specific antibodies. Our data stress that detection of BVDV RNA is not sufficient for a complete risk assessment on FCS. Discrimination between infectious and non-infectious BVDV is essential. This can only be achieved by cell culture methods

Bovine viral diarrhea virus with deletions in the 5'-nontranslated region: reduction of replication in calves and induction of protective immunity
Makoschey, B.; Becher, P.; Janssen, M.G.J.; Orlich, M.; Thiel; H.-J., Lütticken, D.
(2004)
Vaccine 22, 3285-3294

Bovine viral diarrhea virus (BVDV) with deletions in the 5'-nontranslated region (5'-NTR) were tested for their suitability as live BVD vaccines. Firstly, the genetic stability of the mutants was established by culturing over 15 passages in bovine cells. Secondly, two deletion mutants and the parent strain CP7-5A were characterised with respect to in vivo replication competence, attenuation and induction of protective immunity against BVDV. Naive calves (n = 5 per group) were inoculated with mutants d2-31 and d5-57 or CP7-5A and 5 weeks later, a challenge with the BVDV type 1 strain New York was performed. The mutants were found to be genetically and phenotypically stable. Moreover, the results indicate that the mutants were attenuated with regard to effects including pyrexia and drop in leucocyte counts. Infection with the mutants induced moderate to high titers of BVDV neutralizing antibodies and completely prevented viremia after challenge infection with a heterologous BVDV strain. Taken together, the 5'-NTR deletion mutants combine a good safety profile with good efficacy and are therefore well suited as candidate live vaccines

Assessment of the risk of transmission of vaccine viruses by using insufficiently cleaned injection devices
Makoschey, B. and Beer, M. (2004)
The Veterinary Record, 155, 563-564

No abstract available

Comprehensive protection against all important primary pathogens within the bovine respiratory disease complex by combination of two vaccines
Makoschey, B.; Chanter, N.; Reddick, D.A. (2006)
Der praktische Tierarzt 87, 819-826

The compatibility of an inactivated combination vaccine against bovine respiratory syncytial virus (BRSV), bovine parainfluenza type 3 virus (PI3) and Mannheimia haemolytica (*Mh*) with a live IBR marker vaccine was studied. Separate studies were performed to establish the protection against challenge infection with BRSV, PI3, Mh and Bovine herpesvirus type 1 (BoHV-1). The efficacy after single and concurrent administration of the two vaccines was compared. Both vaccination regimes (single and combined vaccine) produced evidence of protection against BRSV and PI3 demonstrated by shorter duration of virus shedding, delayed onset, fewer numbers of animals shedding virus and lower virus titres being recovered. Likewise, concurrent administration of both vaccines resulted in good protection against *Mh* challenge in terms of reduction of clinical signs, lung lesions and lower levels of *Mh* re-isolation from the lungs. Also good protection results against BoHV-1 challenge were obtained. Clinical signs and challenge virus excretion were reduced after vaccination. Most importantly, no differences between single or concurrent administration of the vaccines were determined. In conclusion, the inactivated BRSV / PI3 / Mh combination vaccine and the live IBR marker vaccine tested here were found not to interfere with the efficacy of the different vaccine components. The products can therefore be applied concurrently to prevent infection with all important primary pathogens involved in the bovine respiratory disease complex in one single vaccination measure.

Compatibility of a live Infectious Bovine Rhinotracheitis (IBR) marker vaccine and an inactivated Bovine Viral Diarrhoea Virus (BVDV) vaccine
Álvarez, M.; Muñoz Bielsa, J.; Santos, L.; Makoschey, B. (2007)
Vaccine 25, 6613 - 6617

The target animals and vaccination regimes for vaccines against the bovine rhinotracheitis (IBR) and the bovine viral diarrhoea virus (BVDV) are very similar. Therefore, we have compared different schedules for the combined use of a live IBR marker vaccine and an inactivated BVD vaccine. The neutralizing antibody response against BVDV did not reveal any differences between the group vaccinated only with the BVD vaccine and the groups that were vaccinated simultaneously (together in the same syringe) or concurrently (two separate injections) with the IBR marker vaccine at the first or second dose and the third dose of the BVD vaccine. Likewise, the bovine herpesvirus 1 (BHV-1) neutralizing antibody titres did not exhibit any negative effect by the simultaneous or concurrent use of the two products as compared to the single IBR marker vaccination. These results indicate that the two vaccines can be applied at the same day for the first or second dose of the BVD basic vaccination and then at the booster vaccinations (third dose onwards).

A live bovine herpesvirus-1 marker vaccine is not shed after intramuscular vaccination
Makoschey, B. and Beer, M. (2007)
Berliner und Münchner Tierärztliche Wochenschrift, 120, 480-482

It should be established, whether animals vaccinated intramuscularly (IM) with a live Bovine herpesvirus type 1 (BHV-1) marker vaccine become viremic and/or excrete vaccine virus with nasal discharge. Five cattle, seronegative for BHV-1, were vaccinated with an overdose of the vaccine (Bovilis IBR marker live) via the IM route. Nasal swabs and blood samples were taken at regular intervals and tested for BHV-1 in a virus infectivity assay. In addition, a polymerase chain reaction (PCR) specific for BHV-1 DNA was performed on the blood samples. BHV-1 neutralizing antibody titres were determined in the sera taken prior to the vaccination and four weeks after immunisation. All animals were successfully vaccinated as judged by the development of BHV-1 neutralising antibodies. However, all nasal swab samples were tested negative for vaccine virus, and all blood samples were found negative for BHV-1 vaccine virus and BHV-1 specific DNA. From these data it can be concluded that the vaccine virus was not excreted with nasal discharge after IM vaccination and that the vaccinated animals did not have a detectable viremia. Therefore, it is recommended to apply the tested BHV-1 marker live vaccine by the IM route in situations where it is undesirable that the vaccine virus is excreted.

Evaluation of the induction of NS3 specific BVDV antibodies using a commercial inactivated BVDV vaccine in immunization and challenge trials
Makoschey, B.; Sonnemans, D.; Muñoz Bielsa, J.; Franken, P.; Mars, M.; Santos, L.; Álvarez, M. (2007)
Vaccine 25, 6140 - 6145

In order to evaluate whether cattle vaccinated with an inactivated vaccine against bovine viral diarrhoea virus (BVDV) can be differentiated serologically from BVDV infected animals, two different aspects were investigated. Firstly the antibody response against non-structural proteins (NS) was measured after multiple vaccinations of cattle with a single or double dose of a commercially available inactivated BVDV vaccine. In a second study, the animals were first vaccinated with the product, and then infected with BVDV. The antibody response was determined in four different commercial ELISA systems. It can be concluded, that the inactivated BVD vaccine exhibits properties of a marker vaccine when an appropriate antibody NS3 ELISA is applied: after vaccination NS3-specific antibody levels are low or undetectable, but the vaccination does in the present study not show any interference with the development of antibodies against NS3 after subsequent field virus infection.

Monitoring of a BVDV infection in a vaccinated herd by testing of milk for antibodies against NS3
Kuijk. H.; Franken, P.; Mars, M.; bij de Weg, W.; Makoschey, B. (2008)
The Veterinary Record 163; 482 - 484

No abstract available

Anhang

Submitted for publication:
Development of antibodies against non-structural proteins of the bovine viral diarrhoea virus in serum and milk samples vaccinated animals

Marcelino Álvarez [1], Jorge Donate[2] and Birgit Makoschey[3]*

[1]Department of Animal Health, University of León, Spain
[2]Laboratorios Intervet SA, Salamanca, Spain
[3]Intervet International, Boxmeer, The Netherlands

Corresponding author:
Birgit Makoschey, Intervet International
E-mail: birgit.makoschey@sp.intervet.com

Abstract
Antibodies against the non-structural protein 3 (NS3) of the bovine viral diarrhoea (BVD) virus were determined in milk from cows vaccinated with an inactivated BVD vaccine and compared to serum antibody levels. Animals in one herd were vaccinated with an inactivated BVD vaccine according to the standard protocol and animals from a second herd with an intensive schedule. Serum and milk samples were tested for BVD NS3 antibodies in different commercial tests.
With only a few exceptions, vaccination according to the standard schedule did not induce BVD NS3 antibodies in serum or milk, while such antibodies were detected for a short duration in serum and to a lesser extent in milk after vaccination according to the intensive schedule. Milk was found to be suitable as substrate for BVD monitoring of herds vaccinated with the inactivated BVD vaccine.
Keywords: Bovine viral diarrhoea; marker vaccine; milk test

Introduction
Several EU Member States have already embarked on large scale schemes for the eradication of bovine viral diarrhoea (BVD). The status of these schemes varies a lot with some of them close to finalization and others still in preparation. These schemes have three central elements in common: the implementation of biosecurity, elimination of persistently infected (PI) animals and surveillance (European Thematic Network on Bovine Viral Diarrhoea Virus (BVDV), 2001). The objectives for surveillance are i) to identify PI animals, ii) monitor progress of the interventions and iii) to rapidly detect new infections. Several diagnostic tests are available for the identification of PI animals (Fulton et al., 2006; Hilbe et al., 2007). A diagnostic approach consisting of bulk milk tests for virus and antibody, and antibody tests in samples from young stock is a very useful tool to determine the BVD status of a herd as the results give an indication on the herd prevalence as well as the possible presence of PIs (Mars and Van Maanen, 2005). Once circulation of BVDV in a herd is stopped, milk serological testing of dairy herds is the preferred approach for monitoring of new-infections, both because of time and costs.
In situations where the risk of introducing BVDV infections is high, vaccination can be applied as an additional biosecurity measure (European Thematic Network on Bovine Viral Diarrhoea Virus (BVDV), 2001). A possible issue with the use of BVD vaccines in general could be interference of the antibody response induced by the vaccine with the interpretation of serological test results.

Vaccines that allow differentiation between infected and vaccinated animals, so-called DIVA or marker vaccines would circumvent this problem. To date, no BVDV marker vaccines with specific gene deletions or subunit vaccines are commercialized. A different approach towards a marker vaccine has been followed in case of foot and mouth disease virus. A commercially inactivated vaccine does not induce antibodies against the non-structural protein, (NS) 3ABC, whereas animals infected with field virus typically develop antibodies against this protein (Bruderer et al., 2004). It has been reported earlier that some but not all inactivated BVDV vaccines do not induce detectable antibodies against the NS3 protein (Graham et al., 2003), while animals develop such antibodies after field virus infection. The NS3 protein is a preferred target for commercial BVDV antibody ELISA tests, as the protein is very immunogenic and antibodies against this protein are broadly cross-reacting.
Results from a field study on a Dutch dairy farm indicate that also milk samples are suitable to monitor BVDV infections in vaccinated herds (Kuijk et al., 2008).
The study reported here was performed to further study NS3 antibody response in milk samples after repeated vaccination according to the standard vaccination schedule or an intensive vaccination schedule in a larger number of animals. Moreover, results obtained in milk were compared with the antibody response in serum and compared between different ELISA tests.

Table 1: Time schedule vaccinations and sampling

Group	Number of animals	Vaccinations [days]	Dosing	Sampling
Standard	48 (36*)	0, 28, 208	single	Serum and individual milk: 0, 28, 56, 229
Control (stand)	6	none	None	Tank milk: 0, 28, 56, 208, 229
Intensive single	36 (18*)	0, 28, 56, 84, 112	Single	Serum and individual milk: 0, 28, 56, 84, 112, 140, 168, 196, 240, 330, 426#
Intensive double	20	0, 28, 56, 84, 112	Double	
Control (int)	8	none	none	tank: 0, 28, 56, 84, 112, 140, 168

*available for evaluation of results at the end of the study
if an animal was tested negative in all four tests specific for antibodies against NS3 at day 140 or later, no further samples of serum or milk respectively were taken

Materials and Methods:

Experimental design:
Two separate studies were performed, each in a separate herd. In both studies, animals were vaccinated with a commercial inactivated BVD vaccine or left unvaccinated. In the first study, the vaccinations were performed according to a standard vaccination schedule (two vaccinations at four weeks interval), while in the second study animals were vaccinated 5 times at monthly interval with a single or a double dose of the vaccine or left unvaccinated (see table 1). In both studies serum as well as individual and tank milk samples were taken at the times of vaccination and at pre-set times after the vaccinations. The samples were tested for antibodies.

Experimental animals:
The two studies were performed in two dairy herds, both in the province of Leon (Spain). Both herds were seronegative against BVDV at the start of the study and no animals were introduced into the herds during the course of the study. The herd used for the first study consisted of 54 cows, with 40 cows in lactation at the start of the trial. The second study was performed in a herd of 60 cows with 46 in lactation at the start.

Vaccinations:
All vaccinations were performed with the same inactivated BVD vaccine containing the BVDV-1 strain C86 (Bovilis® BVD, Intervet/Schering-Plough Animal Health). Animals were vaccinated intramuscularly in the neck according to the schedule depicted in table 1.

Sampling and preparation of samples:
Blood and milk samples were taken at the days of vaccination as well as three or four weeks after the vaccination (see table 1). The blood samples were spun at 3.000 rpm during 10 minutes. The serum was collected and stored frozen at temperatures below -20° C until testing.
The milk samples were kept at 4° C for 48 hours. The clotted fat was removed and the milk was collected and stored frozen at temperatures below -20° C until testing.

Table 2: Number of NS3 antibody positive samples (serum and individual milk) or test result (- or + for tank milk) at different time points tested with the different test kits for animals vaccinated according to the standard vaccination schedule (single dose on days 0, 28 and 208)

Date:	Day 0 (1st vacc)			D 28 (2nd vacc)			D 56			D 208 (3rd vacc)	D 229		
Sample:	S*	M	T	S	M	T	S	M	T	T	S	M	T
Test:													
ELISA_A	0	0	-	0	0	-	0	0	-	-	3	2	-
ELISA_B	0	0	-	0	0	-	0	0	-	-	2	1	-
ELISA_C	0	0	-	0	0	-	0	0	-	-	2	1	-
ELISA_D	0	NA#	NA	0	NA	NA	0	NA	NA	NA	2	NA	NA

* S: serum; M: individual milk; T: tank milk
# Only serum samples tested with kit D

Antibody testing:
Antibody response against BVDV NS3 was determined using the following commercial ELISA tests. All these are designed as blocking ELISA.

A) PrioCHECK® BVDV Ab (Prionics, Switzerland). The test was developed as rapid blocking ELISA using two monoclonal antibodies ("WB112" and "WB103") directed to different highly conserved epitopes on the non-structural peptide NS3 of pestiviruses. The ELISA showed a specificity and a sensitivity relative to the virus neutralization test of 99% and 98%, respectively (Kramps et al., 1999b).

B) Pourquier® BVD/MD-BD P80 Ab Blocking ELISA Kit (Pourquier, Montpellier, France). In this ELISA, BVDV antigen is bound to microplates by means of a monoclonal antibody (WB103) specific for the p80 protein of BVDV (Edwards et al., 1988). Serum samples were incubated over night at 4° C. Specific antibodies are quantified by the percentage of blocking the binding of a second monoclonal antibody specific for p80 (WB112) (Edwards et al., 1988).

C) Svanovir® BVDV P80 Ab (Svanova Biotech Ab, Uppsala, Sweden) is a multispecies blocking assay. This test consists of microplates sensitized with the BVD/BD (p80) protein and a peroxidase labelled monoclonal antibody specific for the BVD/BD (p80) protein.

D) INGEZIM BVD COMPAC, (Ingenasa, Madrid, Spain). ELISA plates are coated with BVDV antigen. Specific antibodies are quantified by the percentage of blocking the binding of a second, monoclonal antibody specific for p80 of BVDV, which is not specified in the product information. This test was only used for serum samples.

Antibody response against the whole BVD virus was determined using the following commercial ELISA test:

E) Svanovir® BVDV Ab (Svanova Biotech Ab, Uppsala, Sweden). This test is developed as an indirect ELISA The procedure using 10 microliter of sample was applied. The specificity and sensitivity relative to the virus neutralization for this ELISA are 100% and 98.2%, respectively (Juntti et al., 1987; Svanova Biotech Ab, 2009).

The testing was performed according to the manufacturer's recommendations. In general, serum and milk samples were tested once with the four NS3 ELISAs. In case of inconsistent results, the respective sample was re-tested in duplicate with all four NS3 ELISAs and for each test the results was expressed as average of the three readings for each test.
All tank milk samples were tested in quadruplicates and the average was reported.

Results
Total BVDV antibodies after vaccination
At the beginning of both studies, all animals were seronegative for antibodies against BVDV both in serum and milk. Moreover, all control animals remained seronegative throughout the study.
In the first study, seven animals developed BVDV specific serum antibodies already after the first dose of the vaccine. Three weeks after the second and after the third dose of the vaccine all animals were positive for BVDV specific antibodies in serum. Three weeks after the second dose of vaccine, eight milk samples were found positive, three weeks after the third vaccination, 86% of the available milk samples were found positive (individual data not shown).

In the second study, the seroconversion rates after the first and second vaccination were higher in the serum samples of the animals vaccinated with the double dose (seroconversion rates 50% and 100% after first and second vaccination) regime as compared to the single dose (seroconversion rate 17% and 89% after first and second vaccination) (see Figure 1). From the third dose onwards, all animals in both groups had seroconverted. The milk samples of one animal each in the double and single dose group remained negative throughout the study. Moreover, the development of a positive response in the milk samples was delayed as against the serum samples.

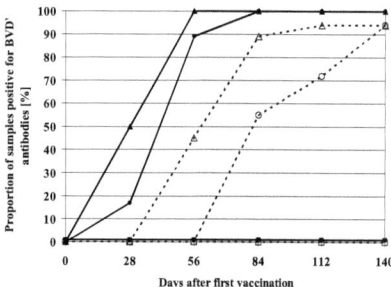

Figure 1: Proportion of serum (—) and milk (---) samples tested positive for BVDV specific antibodies (ELISA_E) after multiple vaccination with a single dose (●,○) or a double dose (▲, △) or left unvaccinated (■, □)

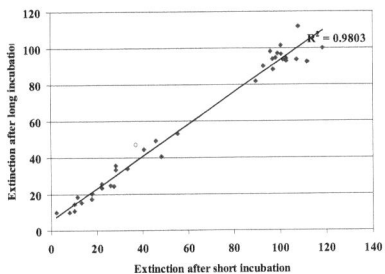

Figure 2: Comparative results for optical density of 37 sera obtained with ELISA_B according to the short (1 hour, 21° C) or the long (over night, 4° C) incubation procedure for serum. (♦) samples that gave the same qualification with both procedures, (○) sample that gave different qualifications with the two procedures

Four weeks after the first vaccination with the double dose regime all samples were still negative and the last animal became only positive after the fourth vaccination. For the animals vaccinated with the single dose regime antibodies were detected in the milk only after the third dose and after the fifth dose 1 animal was still negative for BVDV antibodies.

Comparison of two protocols for sample incubation in ELISA test B

The comparative testing of thirty-seven serum samples according to the short (1 hour, 21° C) and the long (over night, 4° C) incubation procedure gave almost the same results (see fig. 2): There was a very high correlation between the results of the two procedures for the different samples (R^2: 0.9803). With only one exception, the qualification (positive / negative) was identical for both procedures.

Detection of antibodies against BVDV NS3 after vaccination according to the standard schedule

At the beginning of the study, all animals were seronegative for antibodies against BVDV NS3 and all control animals remained seronegative throughout the study. Moreover, animals vaccinated according to the standard schedule were found negative for antibodies specific for BVDV NS3 protein with only a few exceptions on serum and milk samples taken three weeks after the third dose (see table 2). Depending on the assay used, three or two animals were tested positive for serum antibodies and two or one of them were also tested positive for antibodies in milk samples.

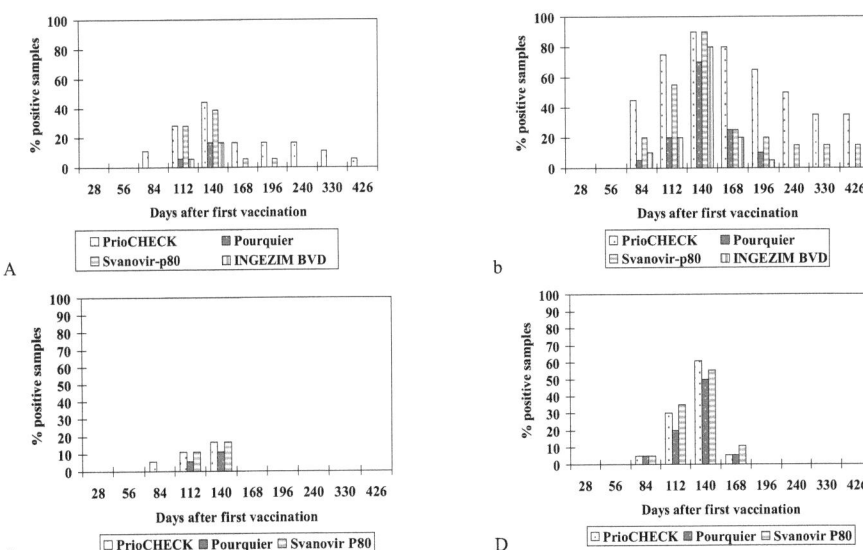

Figure 3: Proportion of positive serum (a, b) and milk (c, d) samples from animals vaccinated according to the intense schedule with the single (a, c) or double (b, d) dose regime, taken at different times after vaccination and tested in the different tests.

Detection of antibodies against BVDV NS3 after vaccination according to the intense schedule

All animals were seronegative for antibodies against BVDV NS3 prior to the first vaccination and all control animals remained seronegative throughout the study. Antibodies against BVDV NS3 proteins were detected in different proportions of the animals vaccinated according to the intense schedule, both in serum and milk samples (see Figure 3). The proportion of positive samples was higher in serum samples as compared to milk. After 5 vaccinations with a single dose only 17% of the animals were positive in milk in at least one test and at least one time point. The repeated (5x) application of a double dose induced BVDV NS specific milk antibodies in 60% of the animals. However, three months after the application of the 5th dose all milk samples were negative.

The bulk milk sample of the herd was tested positive for BVDV NS3 antibodies on day 112 with ELISA_C and on day 140 with ELISA_B (see Table 3). All remaining test results were negative.

Table 3: Results for bulk milk samples of animals vaccinated according to the intense schedule. The results are depicted for the different time points and the different tests.

		Day						
		0	28	56	84	112	140	168
ELISA	A	-	-	-	-	-	-	-
	B	-	-	-	-	-	+	-
	C	-	-	-	-	+	-	-

The distribution of individual results for serum and milk samples from animals vaccinated with the single dose regime according to the intensive schedule are depicted in Figure 4. The results obtained with the various tests followed different patterns: The results on serum with ELISA_A and to a lesser extent also ELISA_C vary within a certain range, which becomes broader with the number of vaccinations. Results obtained with ELISA_B and ELISA_D seem to fall into two categories: The majority of: animals continue to give clearly negative results, while a few animals give positive results after four or five vaccinations. In milk, all three ELISA's gave clearly negative results until after five vaccination for the majority of animals.

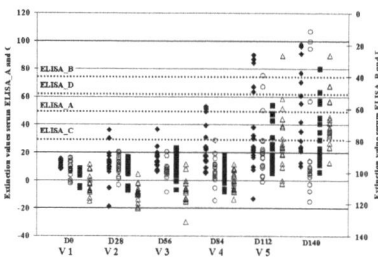

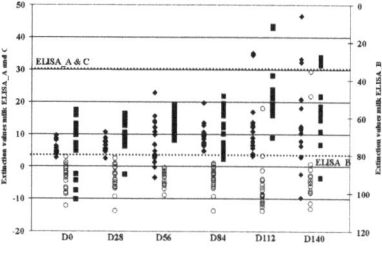

Figure 4: Individual results of serum (a) and milk (b) samples after vaccination with the intensive schedule (single dose) tested by ELISA_A (♦), B (o), C (■) or D (Δ). Values above the threshold (see lines with ELISA name indication) are interpreted as positive.

BVDV NS specific antibody response in milk in relation to the response in serum

As judged by the results obtained in animals vaccinated with the single dose regime according to the intense schedule, there is no direct correlation between the BVDV NS3 specific antibody response measured in milk samples and the result of the respective serum sample (see Figure 5). The regression values were 0.0016, 0.6038, 0.5205 and 0.0712 for ELISA_A, ELISA_B, ELISA_C and ELISA_E respectively.

Discussion:

The response of antibodies against total BVDV in all vaccinated animals confirms that vaccinations have been performed properly. Vaccination according to the standard schedule did not induce serum antibodies against the BVDV NS3 protein in the majority of animals, while such antibodies were detected in samples from animals vaccinated according to the intensive schedule. The proportion of positive animals varied between the different tests and depended on the number of vaccinations and the dosing regime. The antibody response was highest at four weeks after the fifth vaccination and declined sharply during the following months.

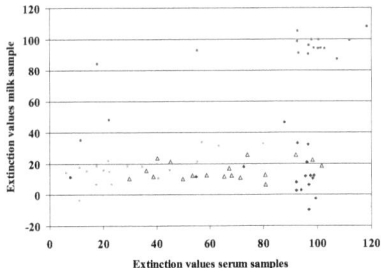

Figure 5: Extinction values for milk samples (study day 140) of animals vaccinated with the single dose regime according to the intensive schedule measured by ELISA_A(●), ELISA_B (♦), ELISA_C (■) and ELISA_E (Δ) in relation to the extinction value for serum samples from the same animal and day.

These observations are in agreement with results obtained in a previous study (Makoschey et al., 2007a).
The apparently very short duration of the NS3 specific immune response is a remarkable observation as the immune response against infection with BVDV is generally considered to be long lasting. Frederiksen and colleagues reported high serum levels of antibodies to BVDV three years after experimental infection (Fredriksen et al., 1999). After vaccination with the same inactivated BVD vaccine used here specific virus neutralising antibodies have been shown to slightly decline with time, but six months after vaccination, titers were still moderate to high (Patel et al., 2002).
In this study, antibody levels in milk were lower than in serum, both for total BVDV and NS3 specific antibodies. Similar results have been reported elsewhere for ELISA_A (Kramps et al., 1999a). However, Bedaudeau and colleagues have fond very similar antibody levels for milk and serum using an ELISA that was not applied in this study (Beaudeau et al., 2001). Evaluation of results from individual matched samples did not show a correlation between antibody levels in serum and milk. Factors other than the serum titer seem to have an influence on the antibody levels in milk. Such factors might be the stage of lactation and the milk yield. The conclusions regarding the comparison of antibody levels in serum and milk do not apply to colostrum, where it has been shown that BVDV antibody titers are higher in colostrum than in serum and antibody levels are correlated (Guerin and Faessel, 2001).
In the study reported here, even after a five vaccinations with a single dose only 17% of the animals were positive in milk in at least one test and at least one time point. Three months after the application of the 5th dose all milk samples, including those from animals that have received the double dose regime were negative again. Moreover, the bulk milk samples of the herd in which the intense vaccination schedule was applied were negative for BVDV NS3 specific antibodies with the exception of two positive test results obtained with different tests on two different sampling days and found negative again one month later and onwards. These results indicate that using milk samples for monitoring of BVDV infection in a herd vaccinated with the inactivated BVDV vaccine used here would result in less "false positive" results than the use of serum samples.
As also described by others (Raue et al., 2008) the results obtained for an individual sample varied between the different tests. Further evaluation of individual results revealed that several samples taken after 5 vaccinations with a single dose gave negative results in ELISA_A and ELISA_C, but the extinction values were actually close to the cut-off level. By contrast, extinction values from serum samples interpreted as negative according to the two blocking ELISAs (ELISA_B and ELISA_D) were clearly beyond the cut-off level (with one exception). Moreover, all three ELISA's applicable for milk gave clearly negative results for the overall majority of samples. Based on these observations, the milk tests seem to be very robust.

Conclusion:
Taken also into consideration previous investigations that the NS3 antibody response of vaccinated and subsequently infected animals followed immunological principles of a booster rather than a primary response (Makoschey et al., 2007b), the results obtained in this study demonstrate that (bulk) milk is a suitable sample for monitoring of BVDV infections in herds vaccinated with the inactivated BVD vaccine used here.
Yet, it should be stressed again that this approach is only suitable for diagnosis on herd level, not for individual animals, as some vaccinated but non-infected animals might develop NS3 specific antibodies shortly after (re-)vaccination and will become seronegative again within a few months.

References
Beaudeau, F., Belloc,C., Seegers,H., Assie,S., Sellal,E.Joly,A., 2001. Evaluation of a blocking ELISA for the detection of bovine viral diarrhoea virus (BVDV) antibodies in serum and milk. Vet. Microbiol. 80, 329-337.

Bruderer, U., Swam,H., Haas,B., Visser,N., Brocchi,E., Grazioli,S., Esterhuysen,J.J., Vosloo,W., Forsyth,M., Aggarwal,N., Cox,S., Armstrong,R.Anderson,J., 2004. Differentiating infection from vaccination in foot-and-mouth-disease: evaluation of an

ELISA based on recombinant 3ABC. Vet. Microbiol. 101, 187-197.

Edwards, S., Sands,J.J.Harkness,J.W., 1988. The application of monoclonal antibody panels to characterize pestivirus isolates from ruminants in Great Britain. Arch. Virol. 102, 197-206.

European Thematic Network on Bovine Viral Diarrhoea Virus (BVDV), 2001. Position Paper BVDV Control in Europe. http://www. bvdv-contro. org.

Fredriksen, B., Sandvik,T., Loken,T.Odegaard,S.A., 1999. Level and duration of serum antibodies in cattle infected experimentally and naturally with bovine virus diarrhoea virus. Vet. Rec. 144, 111-114.

Fulton, R. W., Hessman,B., Johnson,B.J., Ridpath,J.F., Saliki,J.T., Burge,L.J., Sjeklocha,D., Confer,A.W., Funk,R.A.Payton,M.E., 2006. Evaluation of diagnostic tests used for detection of bovine viral diarrhea virus and prevalence of subtypes 1a, 1b, and 2a in persistently infected cattle entering a feedlot. J. Am. Vet. Med. Ass. 228, 578-584.

Graham, D. A., German,A., Mawhinney,K.A.Goodall,E.A., 2003. Antibody responses of naive cattle to two inactivated bovine viral diarrhoea virus vaccines, measured by indirect and blocking ELISA's and virus neutralisation. Vet. Rec. 152, 795-800.

Guerin, G.Faessel,A., 2001. Vaccination with Bovilis BVD at the end of gestation and measurement of anti-BVD antibodies in the colostrum [Vaccination Bovilis BVD en fin de gestation et mesure des titres anticorps anti-BVD dans le colostrum]. Journee Nationales GTV - Cleremont Ferrand 2001 562.

Hilbe, M., Stalder,H., Peterhans,E., Haessig,M., Nussbaumer,M., Egli,C., Schelp,C., Zlinszky,K.Ehrensperger,F., 2007. Comparison of five diagnostic methods for detecting bovine viral diarrhea virus infection in calves. J. Vet. Diagn. Invest. 19, 28-34.

Juntti, N., Larsson,B.Fossum,C., 1987. The use of Monoclonal Antibodies in Enzyme Linked Immunosorbent Assays for Detection of Antibodies to Bovine Viral Diarrhoea Virus. J Vet Med B 34, 356-363.

Kramps, J. A., Van Maanen,C., van de,W.G., Stienstra,G., Quak,S., Brinkhof,J., Ronsholt,L.Nylin,B., 1999a. A simple, rapid and reliable enzyme-linked immunosorbent assay for the detection of bovine virus diarrhoea virus (BVDV) specific antibodies in cattle serum, plasma and bulk milk. Vet. Microbiol. 64, 135-144.

Kramps, J. A., Van Maanen,C., van de,W.G., Stienstra,G., Quak,S., Brinkhof,J., Ronsholt,L.Nylin,B., 1999b. A simple, rapid and reliable enzyme-linked immunosorbent assay for the detection of bovine virus diarrhoea virus (BVDV) specific antibodies in cattle serum, plasma and bulk milk. Vet. Microbiol. 64, 135-144.

Kuijk, H., Franken,P., Mars,M.H., de Weg,W.B.Makoschey,B., 2008. Monitoring of BVDV in a vaccinated herd by testing milk for antibodies to NS3 protein. Vet. Rec. 163, 482-484.

Makoschey, B., Sonnemans,D., Bielsa,J.M., Franken,P., Mars,M., Santos,L.Álvarez,M., 2007b. Evaluation of the induction of NS3 specific BVDV antibodies using a commercial inactivated BVDV vaccine in immunization and challenge trials. Vaccine 25, 6140-6145.

Makoschey, B., Sonnemans,D., Bielsa,J.M., Franken,P., Mars,M., Santos,L.Álvarez,M., 2007a. Evaluation of the induction of NS3 specific BVDV antibodies using a commercial inactivated BVDV vaccine in immunization and challenge trials. Vaccine 25, 6140-6145.

Mars, M. H.Van Maanen,C., 2005. Diagnostic assays applied in BVDV control in The Netherlands. Prev. Vet. Med. 72, 43-48.

Patel, J. R., Shilleto,R.W., Williams,J.Alexander,D.C., 2002. Prevention of transplacental infection of bovine foetus by bovine viral diarrhoea virus through vaccination. Arch. Virol. 147, 2453-2463.

Raue, R., Wright,G.Nanjiani,I.-A., 2008. Comparison of serological response obtained with different bovine viral diarrhea (BVD) ELISA tests after vaccination of young cattle [Comparison de la reponse serologique obtenue avec differents tests ELISA BVD (diarrhee virale bovine) apres vaccination de jeunes bovins. Journee Nationales GTV - Nantes 2008 425-426.

Svanova Biotech Ab, 2009. Product info SVANOVIR BVDV-Ab. http://www.svanova.com/filearchive/BVDV%2007-03.pdf.

Submitted for publication:
Investigations on fetal infection models with bovine viral diarrhoea viruses (BVDV)

B. Makoschey* and M.G.J. Janssen

Intervet/Schering-Plough Animal Health
Wim de Körverstraat 35
3851 AN Boxmeer
The Netherlands

*Corresponding author
Birgit.Makoschey@sp.intervet.com

Summary

Two studies were performed in pregnant heifers to determine whether inoculation of two bovine viral diarrhoea virus (BVDV) strains, one BVDV-1 and one BVDV-2 strain, inoculated separately into either nostril results in fetal infection with both viruses. In a different approach to develop a challenge model for BVDV-2 the efficiency of BVDV-2 transmission from a persistently infected calf to in-contact-cattle was investigated in a third study.
Dual transplacental infection of a fetus with BVDV-1 and BVDV-2 was observed in one occasion but not consistently after concurrent inoculation of both BVDV strains. Transmission of BVDV-2 from PI animals to sentinels was found to be fast and efficient if the animals have direct contact even though they were separated by a fence.

Keywords: Bovine Viral Diarrhoea Virus, Persistent Infection, Transmission, transplacental infection, BVDV

1. Introduction

Bovine viral diarrhoea virus (BVDV) is a major viral pathogen of cattle that has substantial economic importance (Houe 2003). Reproductive disorders account for a major proportion of the economic losses caused by BVDV infection. A key element in the biology and epidemiology of BVDV is the capacity of the virus to cross the placenta and infect the fetus (Fray et al., 2000). Depending on the stage of gestation, this will result in abortion, congenital defects or the birth of a persistently infected (PI) calf. These PI calves are the main source for BVDV transmission within and between cattle herds (Ezanno et al., 2007) and are therefore the key element within BVDV control programs: Programmes in Scandinavian countries that aim at eradicating BVDV without the use of vaccines focus on excluding these PI calves from the market. On the other hand, prevention of fetal infection should be demonstrated for vaccines that are used in BVDV control programs with vaccination (APHIS/USDA 2002; Moennig et al., 2005).
The antigenic and genetic diversity of BVDV has lead to the recognition of two distinct species: BVDV-1 and BVDV-2 (International Committee on Taxonomy of Viruses, ICTV, 2002). While BVDV-1 has been circulating in the cattle population around the world for several decades, BVDV-2 has been first recognized in North America in the 1990s as causative agent of a haemorrhagic syndrome characterized by high fever, thrombocytopenia, haemorrhages and high mortality (Corapi et al., 1990).
Typing of BVDV isolates in samples submitted to the Oklahoma Animal Disease Diagnostic Laboratory revealed that 26% are BVDV-2 (Fulton et al., 2005b). In Europe prevalence of BVDV-2 is low until now (Hurtado et al., 2003; Letellier et al., 1999; Tajima et al., 2001; Wolfmeyer et al., 1997) and some countries with high prevalence of BVDV-1 are reported to be free of BVDV-2 (Stalder et al., 2005).

The aim of the studies reported here was to develop a challenge model for fetal infection with BVDV-2. After simultaneous intranasal inoculation of cattle with BVDV-1 and BVDV-2 dual infection of the fetus with both BVDV species seems to be the exception, rather than the rule (Brock and Chase 2000; Frey et al., 2002; Zimmer et al., 2002). Two studies were performed to investigate whether inoculation of BVDV-1 and BVDV-2 at the same day but into different nostrils leads to a dual infection with both types.

In challenge studies reported in the literature typically several mls of virus suspension at a virus dose between 4 and 7 $\log_{10}TCID_{50}$/ml (Beer et al., 2000; Brock & Chase 2000; Brownlie et al., 1995; Dean and Leyh 1999; Ficken et al., 2006; Frey et al., 2002; Harmeyer et al., 2004; Kovacs et al., 2003; Zimmer et al., 2002) were instilled intranasally at a single occasion. It is generally accepted, that the direct intranasal application of the challenge virus has the advantage of warranting that all animals in the study are exposed to the same virus dose. However, it is difficult to judge, how this approach compares in terms of infectious pressure to the multiple exposure to BVDV shedding from PI calves at a level of about 4-5 $\log_{10}TCID_{50}$/ml under field conditions (Mars et al., 1999). As an alternative to direct intranasal infection, commingling of test animals with PI calves under controlled conditions has been used as well in BVDV challenge studies (Fulton et al., 2005a; Grooms et al., 2007; Patel et al., 2002).

Transmission of BVDV-1 from PIs to in-contact calves has been well studied (Niskanen et al., 2002), however, few information is available, whether BVDV-2 spreads as efficiently as BVDV-1 from PIs to in-contact cattle. Therefore, the third study reported here was performed to determine, whether housing of a PI calf in adjacent pens to the test animals is a reliable model for BVDV-2 vaccination-challenge studies.

2. Materials and Methods

2.1. Viruses and cells

Virus titration, virus isolation and serum neutralization tests were performed on Bovine Embryo Lung (BEL) cells. The cells were cultured in a combination of Glasgow's and Eagles modified minimal essential medium (MEM) supplemented with 5% foetal calf serum and a cocktail of antibiotics neomycin (50µg/ml), polymycin B (50 µg/ml), pimafucin (2.5 µg/ml) and tylosin (10µg/ml). The cells were incubated at 37°C in humidified atmosphere with 5% CO_2.

The noncytopathic BVDV-1 strain CP7 and the noncytopathic BVDV-2 strain Gil have been described before (Becher et al., 1998; Meyers et al., 1996). Inocula for challenge infection were amplified on a proprietary calf kidney cell line (JCK). Aliquots were stored frozen at temperatures below -40°C until use. Prior to the challenge, the viruses were diluted in culture medium. Sterility of all cell and virus stocks was confirmed.

Table 1: Summary of the experimental design of the three animal studies

Study number	Number of animals	Age / duration of pregnancy at challenge	BVDV status	Challenge procedure
Study 1	6	20 months / 2-3 months pregnant	Seronegative / Free of virus	Intranasal inoculation D0
Study 2	5	20 months / 2-3 months pregnant	Seronegative / Free of virus	Intranasal inoculation D0, 1 and 2
Study 3	4	10 months / not pregnant	Seronegative / Free of virus	Contact with PI calf during 4 weeks
	1	3 months / not pregnant	Seronegative / Persistently infected with BVDV-2	Not applicable

2.2. Experimental design of the animal studies

All procedures were approved upfront by the Animal Care and Use Committee according to the Dutch animal welfare regulations.

The experimental design of the three animal studies is summarized in table 1.

Two challenge infection studies were performed in pregnant heifers that were seronegative for BVDV and tested negative for BVDV viremia. At the time of challenge, the heifers were two to three months pregnant. The challenge infection was performed by instillation of 2 ml of the BVDV-1 virus preparation into the right nostril and 2 ml of the BVDV-2 virus preparation in to the left nostril. In the first study, the challenge infection was performed on a single day and the virus content of the inocula was 6.1 $\log_{10}TCID_{50}$ for BVDV-1 and 4.9 $\log_{10}TCID_{50}$ for BVDV-2. In the second study, the animals were inoculated on three consecutive days with the challenge virus preparations and the virus titers were 2.4, 3.3 and 4.5 $\log_{10}TCID_{50}$ of BVDV-1 and 3.2, 4.0 and 5.1 $\log_{10}TCID_{50}$ of BVDV-2 on the first, second and third day respectively.

In both studies, the heifers were monitored for clinical reactions including pyrexia. The clinical parameters were scored as described elsewhere (Makoschey et al., 2001). The method for measuring the neutralising antibody response was described before (Makoschey et al., 2001). The leukocyte and thrombocyte counts were determined. Cell-bound and cell free viremia were measured as described below.

The heifers were followed until the end of pregnancy. Organ samples were taken from aborted fetuses and tested for BVDV (see below). Blood samples were taken from all calves prior to intake of colostrum and tested for BVD virus and specific antibodies. In a third challenge study, four non-pregnant heifers at about 10 months of age were infected by contact with a 3 months old calf that was persistently infected with BVDV-2. The four heifers were housed as one group in a pen, while the PI calf was housed in an adjacent pen. The animals were allowed to have direct contact through the fence. In order to avoid mechanical infection of the in-contact-animals, all handling of the animals was done first with the in-contact-animals and then with the PI calf. Buckets and other materials were not shared between the PI calf and the in-contact- animals. Blood samples were taken weekly from the four heifers and BVDV neutralising antibodies were determined as described (Makoschey et al., 2001).

2.3. Leukocyte and thrombocyte counts

The numbers of circulating leukocytes and thrombocytes were determined using an automated cell counter (Cell-Dyn 3500 hematology analyzer with veterinary software, Abbot). The blood cells were counted according to their size, complexity and depolarization capacity.

2.4. Virus isolation from peripheral blood cells and tissue samples

For the determination of viremia, the buffy coat was recovered as described elsewhere (Makoschey et al., 2001). Aliquots of 10^7 cells were co-cultured in four-fold on monolayers of BEL cells. Sterile samples were taken from aborted foetuses. They were frozen at -70°C until tested for virus by co-culturing with BEL cells.

After 3-5 days of culture the plates were fixated with alcohol, incubated first with an anti-BVDV bovine antiserum and secondly with an anti-bovine FITC-conjugated antibody. The staining was read with a fluorescence microscope.

2.5. Genotyping of BVDV isolates

BVDV isolated from i) selected blood samples of the cows (first study), ii) organ samples from an aborted fetus (first study) or iii) pre-colostral calf sera (second study) were tested by real-time PCR using specific primer sets for BVDV-1 and BVDV-2 as described elsewhere (Makoschey et al., 2003).

3. Results
3.1. Clinical signs and body temperatures of pregnant heifers after infection with BVDV

After infection with BVDV, all heifers developed clinical signs of respiratory disease at varying degree. The signs were judged as mild to moderate, being somewhat more pronounced in the first study than in the second one (See table 2 for individual clinical scores). With the exception of one animal in the second study that had a body temperature of 40°C during one day, no temperatures above 39°C were recorded.

Table 2: Cumulative clinical scores and maximum body temperatures of naïve pregnant heifers during the first two weeks after infection with BVDV.

Study number	Animal number	Clinical scores	Maximum temperature
1	1.1	16	38.6
	1.2	12	38.7
	1.3	9	38.6
	1.4	6	38.7
	1.5	13	38.7
	1.6	4	38.7
2	2.1	5	40.0
	2.2	5	38.9
	2.3	1	38.7
	2.4	3	38.7
	2.5	5	38.7

3.2. Leukocyte counts of pregnant heifers after infection with BVDV

At the time of the infection, leukocyte counts were somewhat higher in the first study (see figure 1). In both studies the numbers of circulating leukocytes started to decrease after the infection of heifers with BVDV. In the first study, normal levels were only reached after more than two weeks post infection, while recovery occurred within less than two weeks in the second study.

3.3. Platelet counts of pregnant heifers after infection with BVDV

Starting four to five days after infection with BVDV, the heifers experienced a drop in platelet counts (see figure 2). In the first study, the platelet counts remained at a low level for several days and normal values were only reached at three weeks after infection. In the second study, the drop recovery took place within a few days.

3.4. BVD viremia of pregnant heifers after infection with BVDV

Prior to the infection all heifers were found to be free of BVD virus. After infection, all heifers were tested positive for BVD viremia for at least one day (see table 3). The viremia peaked around seven or eight days after infection. Most animals were found negative again at two weeks after infection. From the three animals on which a specific PCR was performed, one sample was found positive for BVDV-1 and BVDV-2, while the two other samples were only positive for BVDV-1.

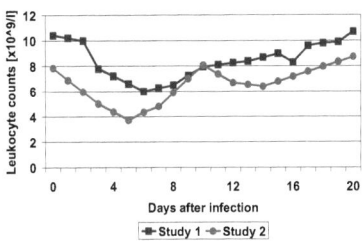

Figure 1: Mean white blood cell counts [x10^9/l] after infection with BVDV-1 and BVDV-2 in the first (■) and second (●) study.

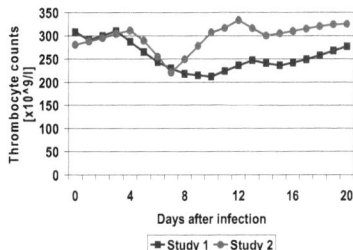

Figure 2: Mean platelet counts [x10^9/l] after infection with BVDV-1 and BVDV-2 in the first (■) and second (●) study.

Table 3: Detection of BVD viremia after infection of naïve pregnant heifers with BVDV.

Study number	Animal number	Day 1st detection	Day last detection	Peak level	BVDV-1 or BVDV-2
1	1.1	8	8	8	#
	1.2	8	10	8	BVDV-1
	1.3	8	15	8	BVDV-1 / BVDV-2
	1.4	6	10	6	#
	1.5	6	10	8	#
	1.6	6	15	6	BVDV-1
2	2.1	7	7	7	#
	2.2	5	7	7	#
	2.3	3	7	7	#
	2.4	3	10	7	#
	2.5	5	7	7	#

BVDV typing was not performed

3.5. Outcome of the pregnancy and BVD viremia in calves born from heifers infected with BVDV during pregnancy

In the first study one heifer aborted six weeks after the infection with BVDV (see table 4). All other pregnancies resulted in the birth of clinically normal calves. One cow in the second study gave birth to twins, all other pregnancies were single calves.

One pre-colostral blood sample taken from a calf in the second study was cytotoxic and therefore, no BVDV could be isolated. All other samples were positive for BVDV. Likewise, BVDV could be isolated from the organ samples of the aborted fetus. In the latter samples, BVDV-1 and BVDV-2 was detected by specific PCR, while only BVDV-2 was detected in the calves' serum samples from study two. (Specific PCR was not performed on blood samples from calves born in the first study).

3.6. Neutralising antibody response after infection of pregnant heifes with BVDV

At the time of infection all heifers were seronegative for BVDV-1 and BVDV-2 (see figure 3a and 3b for the first and second study respectively). At one month after the infection, all heifers had developed antibodies against BVDV-1 and BVDV-2. In the first study, titers continued to increase during the following months until the end of the study at 6 months after infection. In the second study, titers increased between one and three months after infection but thereafter they remained rather stable until the end of the study.

Overall, titers against BVDV-2 were higher than against BVDV-1 and with a few exceptions, the courses of antibody titers of an animal against both titers run in parallel. Exceptions are animal number five in the first study (identification number 1.5) that has stable titers against BVDV-2 between 4 and 6 months after infection, while the titers against BVDV-1 are increasing during the same period and animal number four in the second study (identification number 2.4) that has higher titers against BVDV-1 at 1 months after infection.

3.7. Neutralising antibody response and clinical signs of naive heifers after contact with BVDV PI calf

At the time of introduction of the PI animal, the four heifers were seronegative for BVDV (see figure 4) and they all remained seronegative until two weeks after introduction of the PI calf. Three weeks after the introduction of the PI animal, three out of the four in-contact-animals developed antibodies against BVDV and the fourth animal seroconverted during the following week. None of the in-contact-animals developed clinical signs.

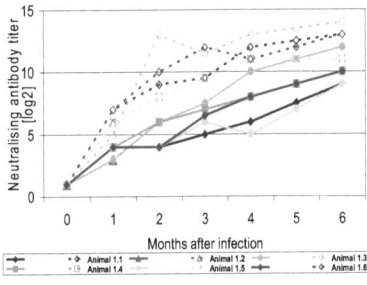 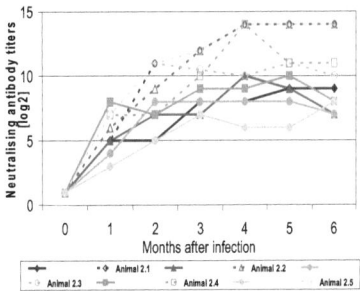

Fig 3: Individual neutralising antibody response against BVDV-1 (solid symbols) and BVDV-2 (empty symbols) in the first (a) and second (b) study

4. Discussion

Only mild to moderate clinical sings were observed in both studies after intranasal inoculation of pregnant heifers with BVDV-1 and BVDV-2 and BVDV infection occurred clinically unnoticed in the third study. The variation in acute virulence between BVDV strains is generally accepted (Ridpath et al., 2007). Both strains were used in previous studies to infect calves under experimental conditions: While the cytopathic (cp) biotype of the BVDV-1 strain CP7 has induced pyrexia but only mild clinical signs (Makoschey et al., 2004), clinical signs of respiratory disease and diarrhoea have been observed in calves at the age of 20 weeks after infection with the cp / ncp pair of the same BVDV-2 strain (Gil) used here (Makoschey et al., 2001). The discrepancy between the clinical signs observed in calves after infection with the BVDV-2 strain Gil and the two studies in pregnant heifers can have different reasons. The age might be an important factor in this respect as also under field conditions infection with BVDV in adult cattle often passes without obvious clinical disease (Ames 1986; Moerman et al., 1994). Another difference between the study in calves and those in heifers is the virus dose which was considerably higher in the calves. However, reports on the effect of the virus dose on the severity of clinical presentation are controversial (Polak and Zmudzinski 2000; Ridpath et al., 2007). The third difference is the use of both biotypes of the BVDV-2 strain Gil in the calves study, whereas the pregnant heifers were only infected with the ncp biotype as there is no evidence that infection *in utero* with cytopathic virus results in a persistent viremia (Brownlie et al., 1989). Unpublished results of an earlier study indicated that the pathogenicity of the BDV-2 challenge strain was related to the cp virus.

Interestingly, the reduction of circulating white blood cells observed in the two studies in pregnant heifers was very similar to the data obtained after infection of calves with either of the two BVDV challenge viruses. During an acute BVDV infection, not only the number of lymphocytes is reduced (Bolin et al., 1985), but the virus is also known to interfere at different levels with the innate immunity (Peterhans et al., 2003), which then often facilitates secondary infections. The degree of lymphocyte depletion was comparable between the two studies in pregnant heifers, though in the first trial the absolute numbers of lymphocytes were higher throughout the whole study and the recovery in lymphocyte counts was delayed as compared to the second trial. Also the depression in thrombocyte counts was of shorter duration in the second study as compared to the first one. This may indicate that the challenge in the first trial was somehow more severe than in the second trial.

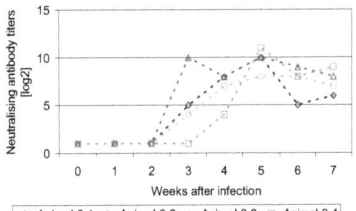

Fig 4: Individual neutralising antibody response against BVDV-2 of naive cattle after contact with a BVDV-2 persistently infected calf

Table 4: Outcome of the pregnancy and detection of BVD virus in pre-colostral calf sera

Study number	Animal identification number	Number of live / dead calves	Detection of BVDV precolostral sera	Detection of BVDV organs	Typing of BVDV isolated from calf / fetus
1	1.1	1/0	+	-	#
	1.2	0/1	-	+	BVDV-1 and BVDV-2
	1.3	1/0	+	-	#
	1.4	1/0	+	-	#
	1.5	1/0	+	-	#
	1.6	1/0	+	-	#
2	2.1	1/0	+	-	BVDV-2
	2.2	1/0	+	-	BVDV-2
	2.3	1/0	*	-	
	2.4	1/0	+	-	BVDV-2
	2.5	2/0	+	-	BVDV-2
			+	-	BVDV-2

* No virus isolated due to toxic effect of sample
# BVDV typing was not performed on pre-colostral blood samples

The most obvious difference between both studies was the challenge procedure. In the second study the animals were inoculated on three subsequent days with increasing virus doses. The BVDV-1 virus dose applied on the third day was 40 times lower than the dose applied in the first study. For BVDV-2 the dose on the third challenge day of the second study was comparable to the dose inoculated in the first study. On the first or second day the challenge doses were considerably lower than in the first study. If the animals became already infected by the lower challenge virus doses it is likely that they were refractory to the higher doses on the following days. Under field conditions PI animals shed BVDV at a level of about 4-5 $\log_{10}TCID_{50}$/ml (Mars et al., 1999), however in-contact animals will often be exposed to rather small volumes of nasal discharge. Therefore, the virus doses used on the first and second day of challenge in the second study might reflect the situation of virus transmission from a PI animal.
Thrombocytopenia was a predominant finding in the first reports on BVDV-2 outbreaks with haemorrhagic disease (Corapi et al., 1990; Rebhun et al., 1989), however, more recently thrombocytopenia has also been described after infection with virulent BVDV-1 strains (Ridpath et al., 2007). Therefore it is not justified to speculate based on the decrease in platelet counts in all heifers in the two studies reported here (individual data not show) that they were infected with BVDV-2.
Overall the pregnant heifers developed higher titers against BVDV-2 as compared to BVDV-1. The capacity to induce cross-neutralising antibodies varies between BVDV isolates and it has been shown before that BVDV-2 strain Gil induces a strong cross-neutralising antibody response also against BVDV-1 strains (Patel et al., 2005). In general, the courses of antibody titers against BVDV-1 and BVDV-2 ran in parallel, making it difficult to judge whether the animals were infected with a single virus or both viruses. Only in two animals (1.5 and 2.4) the difference in the course of antibody titers against BVDV-1 and BVDV-2 was indicative for a separate infection with both viruses at different time points.

Table 5: BVDV neutralizing antibody titers against BVDV type 2 strain 890 [$\log_2$]

Animal	T=0	t=1 week	t=2 weeks	T=3 weeks	t=4 weeks	t=5 weeks	T=6 weeks	t=7 weeks
1	<2	<2	<2	5	8	10	5	6
2	<2	<2	<2	10	8	10	9	8
3	<2	<2	<2	4	7	8	8	7
4	<2	<2	2*	<2	4	11	8	9

▲Titer of <2 considered negative; * unspecific reaction (next sample is negative)

In the first study virus re-isolated from 3 heifers was typed by RT-PCR and BVDV-1 was found in all three isolates and in addition BVDV-2 in one of them. Interestingly BVDV-1 and BVDV-2 were isolated from a calf born from one of the two heifers from which only BVDV-1 was detected. Most likely viremia of the two BVDV strains did not follow the same time course in that heifer.

The detection of BVDV-1 and BVDV-2 genome sequences in one calf born in the first study confirmed that dual infection of the fetus is possible under experimental conditions (Brock & Chase 2000; Zimmer et al., 2002). However, this result could not be reproduced in the second study, where only BVDV-2 was detected in the calves. It has been reported before that only one BVDV isolate was detected in most or all calves from mothers that have been inoculated with a mixture of two or more BVDV strains (Brock & Chase 2000; Frey et al., 2002; Zimmer et al., 2002). Differing from those studies, the two BVDV strains were instilled separately into the left and right nostril in the studies reported here. This approach was chosen to avoid competition for target cells at the site of primary virus replication in the lymphoid tissues lining the oropharynx (Bielefeldt-Ohmann 1983). However, also after separate inoculation of the two BVDV challenge virus strains dual infection of the fetus could not be reproduced consistently. The most obvious explanation would be that after infection with two or more BVDV strains only one can establish a systemic infection, even after instillation into different nostrils. However experimental data on modified live BVDV-1 and BVDV-2 combination vaccines (Ellsworth et al., 2006; Endsley et al., 2002; Shelton et al., 2006) supported by experiences from use in the field have shown that the two vaccine viruses establish a solid immune response indicative for replication of both vaccine viruses in the immunized animal.

Since dual fetal infection with BVDV-1 and BVDV-2 could not be achieved consistently after intranasal inoculation, separate challenge studies for either BVDV species might be required.

Commingling of test animals with PI animals under controlled conditions (Fulton et al., 2005a; Grooms et al., 2007; Patel et al., 2002) mimics the circumstances of natural infections. As for any other challenge model, infection of all control animals is a basic requirement. Transmission of BVDV-1 from PI animals to in-contact calves has been achieved in 100% (Niskanen et al., 2000; Patel et al., 2002) or 83% (Fulton et al., 2005a) of the animals.

In the study reported here all in-contact animals were successfully infected with BVDV-2. The antibody responses of the individual animals indicate that the infection took place in the first two weeks after first contact with the PI animal.

These results point to a transmission of BVDV-2 from PI animals is as efficient as for BVDV-1. In this perspective it is very remarkable that the prevalence of BVDV-2 in Europe is still much lower than BVDV-1 (Hurtado et al., 2003; Letellier et al., 1999; Stalder et al., 2005; Tajima et al., 2001; Wolfmeyer et al., 1997), despite the fact that vaccines against BVDV-1 but not BVDV-2 are widely used.

Based on the experimental data reported here, and similar findings by others for BVDV-1 (McGowan et al., 1993; Meyling and Jensen 1988), one would expect, that most herds with contact to a PI animal display seroconversion rates close to 100%. However, in general, infection rates determined under field conditions, are lower (Beaudeau et al., 2001; Fulton et al., 2005a; Mawhinney et al., 2007). A possible explanation for this discrepancy might be the smaller number of animals and the smaller size of the stables in the experimental studies as compared to average herd sizes in the field. These two factors are directly related to the probability of direct animal to animal contacts. Airborne transmission of BVDV from PI animals to sentinel calves has been demonstrated (Mars et al., 1999), however, direct animal-to-animal contact seems to be the most efficient and predominant mode of transmission. This might also explain, why seroconversion rates can be vary between different housing groups in a herd (Mawhinney et al., 2007).

5. Conclusions

In conclusion, the data reported here demonstrate, that concurrent infection of pregnant cattle with two BVDV strains does not consistently result in dual transplacental infection of the fetuses. In a separate approach to develop a BVDV-2 challenge model, transmission of BVDV-2 from PI animals to sentinels has been shown to be fast and efficient if the animals have direct contact, even if they are separated by a fence.

6. Acknowledgement

The authors are most grateful to the colleagues from the Animal Service Department, especially Marianne Smit and Henk Zwinkels, for their excellent technical assistance and dedicated care for the calves.

7. References

Ames, T.R., 1986. The causative agent of BVD: Its epidemiology and pathogenesis. Veterinary Medicine **81**, 848-869.

APHIS/USDA, 2002. CVB notice 02-1919 Vaccine Claims for Protection of the Fetus against BVDV. In: Biologicals/APHIS/USDA CfV.

Beaudeau, F., Assie, S., Seegers, H., Belloc, C., Sellal, E., Joly, A., 2001. Assessing the within-herd prevalence of cows antibody-positive to bovine viral diarrhoea virus with a blocking ELISA on bulk tank milk. The Veterinary Record **149**, 236-240.

Becher, P., Orlich, M., König, M., Thiel, H.-J., 1998. Nonhomologous RNA recombination in bovine viral diarrhea virus: Molecular characterization of a variety of subgenomic RNAs isolated during an outbreak of fatal mucosal disease. Journal of Virology **73**, 5646-5653.

Beer, M., Hehnen, H.R., Wolfmeyer, A., Poll, G., Kaaden, O.-R., Wolf, G., 2000. A new inactivated BVDV genotype I and II vaccine An immunisation and challenge study with BVDV genotype I. Veterinary Microbiology **77**, 195-208.

Bielefeldt-Ohmann, H., 1983. Pathogenesis of bovine viral diarrhoea-mucosal disease: distribution and significance of BVDV antigen in diseased calves. Research in Veterinary Science **34**, 5-10.

Bolin, S.R., McClurkin, A.W., Coria, M.F., 1985. Effects of Bovine Viral Diarrhea Virus on the Percentages and Absolute Numbers of Circulating B and T Lymphocytes in Cattle. American Journal of Veterinary Research **46 (4)**, 884-886.

Brock, K.V., Chase, C.C., 2000. Development of a fetal challenge method for the evaluation of bovine viral diarrhea virus vaccines. Veterinary Microbiology **77**, 209-214.

Brownlie, J., Clarke, M.C., Hooper, L.B., Bell, G.D., 1995. Protection of the bovine fetus from bovine viral diarrhoea virus by means of a new inactivated vaccine. The Veterinary Record **137**, 58-62.

Brownlie, J., Clarke, M.C., Howard, C.J., 1989. Experimental infection of cattle in early pregnancy with a cytopathic strain of bovine virus diarrhoea virus. Research in Veterinary Science **46**, 307-311.

Corapi, W.V., Elliott, R.D., French, T.W., Arthur, D.G., Bezek, D.M., Dubovi, E., 1990. Thrombocytopenia and hemorrhages in veal calves infected with bovine viral diarrhea virus. Journal of American Veterinary Medicine Association **196**, 590-596.

Dean, H.J., Leyh, R., 1999. Cross-protective efficacy of a bovine viral diarrhea virus (BVDV) type 1 vaccine against BVDV type 2 challenge. Vaccine **17**, 1117-1124.

Ellsworth, M.A., Fairbanks, K.K., Behan, S., Jackson, J.A., Goodyear, M., Oien, N.L., Meinert, T.R., Leyh, R.D., 2006. Fetal protection following exposure to calves persistently infected with bovine viral diarrhea virus type 2 sixteen months after primary vaccination of the dams. Veterinary Therapy **7**, 295-304.

Endsley, J.J., Quade, M.J., Terhaar, B., Roth, J.A., 2002. Bovine viral diarrhea virus type 1- and type 2-specific bovine T lymphocyte-subset responses following modified-live virus vaccination. Veterinary Therapy **3**, 364-372.

Ezanno, P., Fourichon, C., Viet, A.F., Seegers, H., 2007. Sensitivity analysis to identify key-parameters in modelling the spread of bovine viral diarrhoea virus in a dairy herd. Preventive Veterinary Medicine **80**, 49-64.

Ficken, M.D., Ellsworth, M.A., Tucker, C.M., Cortese, V.S., 2006. Effects of modified-live bovine viral diarrhea virus vaccines containing either type 1 or types 1 and 2 BVDV on heifers and their offspring after challenge with noncytopathic type 2 BVDV during gestation. Journal of American Veterinary Medicine Association **228**, 1559-1564.

Fray, M.D., Paton, D.J., Alenius, S., 2000. The effects of bovine viral diarrhoea virus on cattle reproduction in relation to disease control. Animal Reproduction Science **60-61**, 615-627.

Frey, H.R., Eicken, K., Grummer, B., Kenklies, S., Oguzoglu, T.C., Moennig, V., 2002. Foetal protection against bovine virus diarrhoea virus after two-step vaccination. Journal of Veterinary Medicine B **49**, 489-493.

Fulton, R.W., Briggs, R.E., Ridpath, J.F., Saliki, J.T., Confer, A.W., Payton, M.E., Duff, G.C., Step, D.L., Walker, D.A., 2005a. Transmission of bovine viral diarrhea virus 1b to susceptible and vaccinated calves by exposure to persistently infected calves. Canadian Journal of Veterinary Research **69**, 161-169.

Fulton, R.W., Ridpath, J.F., Ore, S., Confer, A.W., Saliki, J.T., Burge, L.J., Payton, M.E., 2005b. Bovine viral diarrhoea virus (BVDV) subgenotypes in diagnostic laboratory accessions: distribution of BVDV1a, 1b, and 2a subgenotypes. Veterinary Microbiology **111**, 35-40.

Grooms, D.L., Bolin, S.R., Coe, P.H., Borges, R.J., Coutu, C.E., 2007. Fetal protection against continual exposure to bovine viral diarrhea virus following administration of a vaccine containing an inactivated bovine viral diarrhea virus fraction to cattle. American Journal of Veterinary Research **68**, 1417-1422.

Harmeyer, S.S., Antonis, A.F., Gadd, T., Salt, J.S., Jahnecke, S., Brune, A., 2004. Fetal protection against BVDV fetal infection six months after vaccination with a novel BVDV vaccine (Schutz vor transplazentarer Infektion mit BVDV nach Impfung mit einer neuen inaktivierten BVD-Vakzine (PregSure® BVD)). Tierärztliche Umschau **59**, 663-668.

Houe, H., 2003. Economic impact of BVDV infection in dairies. Biologicals **31**, 137-143.

Hurtado, A., Garcia-Perez, A.L., Aduriz, G., Juste, R.A., 2003. Genetic diversity of ruminant pestiviruses from Spain. Virus Research **92**, 67-73.

Kovacs, F., Magyar, T., Rinehart, C., Elbers, K., Schlesinger, K., Ohnesorge, W.C., 2003. The live attenuated bovine viral diarrhea virus components of a multi-valent vaccine confer protection against fetal infection. Veterinary Medicine **96**, 117-131.

Letellier, C., Kerkhofs, P., Wellemans, G., Vanopdenbosch, E., 1999. Detection and genotyping of bovine diarrhea virus by reverse transcription-polymerase chain amplification of the 5' untranslated region. Veterinary Microbiology **64**, 155-167.

Makoschey, B., Becher, P., Janssen, M.G., Orlich, M., Thiel, H.J., Lutticken, D., 2004. Bovine viral diarrhea virus with deletions in the 5'-nontranslated region: reduction of replication in calves and induction of protective immunity. Vaccine **22**, 3285-3294.

Makoschey, B., Janssen, M.G., Vrijenhoek, M.P., Korsten, J.H., Marel, P., 2001. An inactivated bovine virus diarrhoea virus (BVDV) type 1 vaccine affords clinical protection against BVDV type 2. Vaccine **19**, 3261-3268.

Makoschey, B., van Gelder, P.T., Keijsers, V., Goovaerts, D., 2003. Bovine viral diarrhoea virus antigen in foetal calf serum batches and consequences of such contamination for vaccine production. Biologicals **31**, 203-208.

Mars, M.H., Bruschke, C.J., van Oirschot, J.T., 1999. Airborne transmission of BHV1, BRSV, and BVDV among cattle is possible under experimental conditions. Veterinary Microbiology **66**, 197-207.

Mawhinney, I., Watson, C., Patel, J.R., 2007. Seroprevalence of BVDV in cattle of different age groups on 17 dairy farms in the West of England. The Veterinary Record **160**, 738-740.

McGowan, M.R., Kirkland, P.D., Richards, S.G., Littlejohns, I.R., 1993. Increased reproductive losses in cattle infected with bovine pestivirus around the time of insemination. The Veterinary Record **133**, 39-43.

Meyers, G., Tautz, N., Becher, P., Thiel, H.J., Kümmerer, B.M., 1996. Recovery of cytopathogenic and noncytopathogenic bovine viral diarrhea viruses from cDNA constructs. Journal of Virology **70**, 8606-8613.

Meyling, A., Jensen, A.M., 1988. Transmission of bovine virus diarrhoea virus (BVDV) by artificial insemination (AI) with semen from a persistently-infected bull. Veterinary Microbiology **17**, 97-105.

Moennig, V., Houe, H., Lindberg, A., 2005. BVD control in Europe: current status and perspectives. Anim Health Research Review **6**, 63-74.

Moerman, A., Straver, P.J., De Jong, M.C., Quak, J., Baanvinger, T., van Oirschot, J.T., 1994. Clinical consequences of a bovine virus diarrhoea virus infection in a dairy herd: a longitudinal study. Veterinary Quarterly **16**, 115-119.

Niskanen, R., Lindberg, A., Larsson, B., Alenius, S., 2000. Lack of virus transmission from bovine viral diarrhoea virus infected calves to susceptible peers. Acta Veterinaria Scandinavia **41**, 93-99.

Niskanen, R., Lindberg, A., Traven, M., 2002. Failure to spread bovine virus diarrhoea virus infection from primarily infected calves despite concurrent infection with bovine coronavirus. The Veterinary Journal **163**, 251-259.

Patel, J.R., Didlick, S., Quinton, J., 2005. Variation in immunogenicity of ruminant pestiviruses as determined by the neutralisation assay. The Veterinary Journal **169**, 468-472.

Patel, J.R., Shilleto, R.W., Williams, J., Alexander, D.C., 2002. Prevention of transplacental infection of bovine foetus by bovine viral diarrhoea virus through vaccination. Archives of Virology **147**, 2453-2463.

Peterhans, E., Jungi, T.W., Schweizer, M., 2003. BVDV and innate immunity. Biologicals **31**, 107-112.

Polak, M.P., Zmudzinski, J.F., 2000. Experimental inoculation of calves with laboratory strains of bovine viral diarrhea virus. Comparitive Immunology Microbiology and Infectious Diseases. **23,** 141-151.

Rebhun, W.C., French, T.W., Perdrizet, J.A., Dubovi, E., Dill, S.G., Karcher, L.F., 1989. Thrombocytopenia associated with acute bovine virus diarrhea infection in cattle. Journal of Veterinary Internal Medicine **3,** 42-46.

Ridpath, J.F., Neill, J.D., Peterhans, E., 2007. Impact of variation in acute virulence of BVDV1 strains on design of better vaccine efficacy challenge models. Vaccine **25,** 8058-8066.

Shelton, T., Xue, W., Makoschey, B., 2006. Protection against fetal persistent infection (PI) caused by BVDV type 1 and BVDV type 2 for a single vaccination with a multivalent modified live vaccine pre-breeding. 25th World Buiatrics Congress 2006, Nice, Oct 15-19 2006.

Stalder, H.P., Meier, P., Pfaffen, G., Wageck-Canal, C., Rufenacht, J., Schaller, P., Bachofen, C., Marti, S., Vogt, H.R., Peterhans, E., 2005. Genetic heterogeneity of pestiviruses of ruminants in Switzerland. Preventive Veterinary Medicine **72,** 37-41.

Tajima, M., Frey, H., Yamato, O., Maede, Y., Moennig, V., Scholz, H., Greiser-Wilke, I., 2001. Prevalence of genotypes 1 and 2 of bovine viral diarrhea virus in Lower Saxony, Germany. Virus Research **76,** 31-42.

Wolfmeyer, A., Wolf, G., Beer, M., Strube, W., Hehnen, H.R., Schmeer, N., Kaaden, O.-R., 1997. Genomic (5'UTR) and serological differences among Germany BVDV field isolates. Archives of Virology **142,** 2049-2057.

Zimmer, G.M., Wentink, G.H., Bruschke, C., Westenbrink, F.J., Brinkhof, J., de, G., I, 2002. Failure of foetal protection after vaccination against an experimental infection with bovine virus diarrhea virus. Veterinary Microbiology **89,** 255-265.

SINGLE VACCINATION WITH AN INACTIVATED BOVINE RESPIRATORY SYNCYTIAL VIRUS VACCINE PRIMES THE CELLULAR IMMUNE RESPONSE IN CALVES WITH MATERNAL ANTIBODY

van der Sluijs, M.T.W., Kuhn, E.M. and Makoschey, B. (2010)
BMC veterinary research 6(1):2 [The article was published after submission of the habilitation script]

Background: The efficacy of a single dose of an inactivated bovine respiratory syncytial virus (BRSV) - Parainfluenaza type 3 (PI3) – *Mannheimia haemolytica* (*Mh*) combination vaccine, in calves positive for maternal antibodies, was established in a BRSV infection study.
Results: As expected the single vaccination did not have any effect on the decline of BRSV-specific neutralising or ELISA antibody. The cellular immune system was however primed by the vaccination. In the vaccinated group virus excretion with nasal discharge was reduced, less virus could be re-isolated from lung tissues and the lungs were less affected.
Conclusions: These results indicate that a single vaccination with an inactivated BRSV vaccine was able to break through the maternal immunity and induce partial protection in very young calves. It can be speculated that the level and duration of protection will improve after the second dose of vaccine is administered. A two-dose basic vaccination schedule is recommended under field conditions

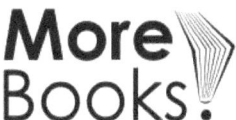

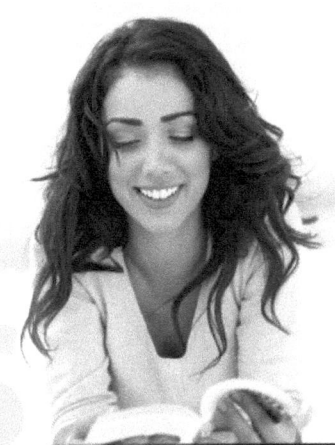

I want morebooks!

Buy your books fast and straightforward online - at one of world's fastest growing online book stores! Environmentally sound due to Print-on-Demand technologies.

Buy your books online at
www.morebooks.shop

Kaufen Sie Ihre Bücher schnell und unkompliziert online – auf einer der am schnellsten wachsenden Buchhandelsplattformen weltweit! Dank Print-On-Demand umwelt- und ressourcenschonend produziert.

Bücher schneller online kaufen
www.morebooks.shop

KS OmniScriptum Publishing
Brivibas gatve 197
LV-1039 Riga, Latvia
Telefax: +371 686 204 55

info@omniscriptum.com
www.omniscriptum.com

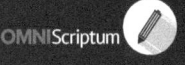

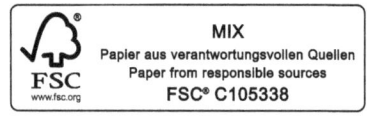

Printed by Books on Demand GmbH, Norderstedt / Germany